Psychiatric Expert Testimony: Emerging Applications

PSYCHIATRIC EXPERT TESTIMONY: EMERGING APPLICATIONS

Edited by Kenneth J. Weiss, MD

and

Clarence Watson, JD, MD

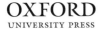

OXFORD
UNIVERSITY PRESS

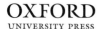

Oxford University Press is a department of the University of
Oxford. It furthers the University's objective of excellence in research,
scholarship, and education by publishing worldwide.

Oxford   New York
Auckland   Cape Town   Dar es Salaam   Hong Kong   Karachi
Kuala Lumpur   Madrid   Melbourne   Mexico City   Nairobi
New Delhi   Shanghai   Taipei   Toronto

With offices in
Argentina   Austria   Brazil   Chile   Czech Republic   France   Greece
Guatemala   Hungary   Italy   Japan   Poland   Portugal   Singapore
South Korea   Switzerland   Thailand   Turkey   Ukraine   Vietnam

Oxford is a registered trademark of Oxford University Press
in the UK and certain other countries.

Published in the United States of America by
Oxford University Press
198 Madison Avenue, New York, NY 10016

Library of Congress Cataloging-in-Publication Data
Psychiatric expert testimony : emerging applications / edited by Kenneth J. Weiss,
Clarence Watson.
    p.; cm.
Includes bibliographical references and index.
ISBN 978–0–19–934659–2 (alk. paper)
ISBN 978–0–19–934660–8 (updf)
ISBN 978–0–19–934661–5 (epub)
I. Weiss, Kenneth J. editor.   II. Watson, Clarence, editor. [DNLM: 1. Forensic Psychiatry—
United States.   2. Brain—pathology—United States.   3. Criminal Law—United
States.   4. Criminals—psychology—United States.   5. Expert Testimony—United States.
W 740] RA1148 614.15—dc23
2014022899

This material is not intended to be, and should not be considered, a substitute for medical or other
professional advice. Treatment for the conditions described in this material is highly dependent on
the individual circumstances. And, while this material is designed to offer accurate information
with respect to the subject matter covered and to be current as of the time it was written, research
and knowledge about medical and health issues is constantly evolving and dose schedules for
medications are being revised continually, with new side effects recognized and accounted for
regularly. Readers must therefore always check the product information and clinical procedures
with the most up-to-date published product information and data sheets provided by the
manufacturers and the most recent codes of conduct and safety regulation. The publisher and the
authors make no representations or warranties to readers, express or implied, as to the accuracy or
completeness of this material. Without limiting the foregoing, the publisher and the authors make
no representations or warranties as to the accuracy or efficacy of the drug dosages mentioned in the
material. The authors and the publisher do not accept, and expressly disclaim, any responsibility
for any liability, loss or risk that may be claimed or incurred as a consequence of the use and/or
application of any of the contents of this material.

9 8 7 6 5 4 3 2 1
Printed in the United States of America
on acid-free paper

CONTENTS

FOREWORD

BY ROBERT L. SADOFF

The field of forensic psychiatry has grown significantly during the past half-century. Rising from the few physicians who were referred to as *alienists* in the 19th century, forensic psychiatry has become one of the major subspecialties of psychiatry. Spurred by the inauguration of the American Academy of Psychiatry and the Law in 1969, the field has burgeoned to include a number of major professional organizations, scientific journals, and scores of textbooks. Under the leadership of Dr. Richard Rosner, fellowship training in forensic psychiatry began in the 1980s and has led to a current 40 ACGME-accredited training programs in forensic psychiatry throughout the country. Board certification in forensic psychiatry began with the American Board of Forensic Psychiatry, and currently certification is authorized under the aegis of the American Board of Psychiatry and Neurology.

Forensic psychiatry is but one of the many forensic sciences that are essential to modern-day court cases in which scientific evidence is presented in both civil and criminal cases. Standards for presenting expert psychiatric testimony have developed through legislation, case law, and professional organizations. The judge is the gatekeeper to prevent "junk science" from being presented at trial, and rules have been developed to limit the testimony of various professionals. In addition, professional organizations have developed ethical guidelines under which their members must testify.

As the use of forensic specialists has grown, so has the need for training and education in the emerging issues that confront the expert testifying in court. Drs. Weiss and Watson have assembled a group of authors to illustrate the emerging issues for the forensic psychiatric expert. Dr. Weiss is a senior forensic psychiatrist who has developed an expertise in the history of medicine, psychiatry, and forensic psychiatry. Dr. Watson, who is also an attorney, has used his integrative education to improve his skills in the field.

As the editors point out, most cases do not go to trial but are settled. The forensic psychiatrist has multiple roles to play in civil and criminal cases aside from testifying in court. The 4 major efforts by the forensic psychiatrist are examining the plaintiff or defendant, writing a report, consulting with attorneys, and testifying either at deposition or at trial. Increasingly, the role of the forensic psychiatrist has become that of a consultant to the lawyer or at times to the court. The forensic psychiatrist may use his or her educational skills in teaching lawyers, judges, or even juries emerging issues that need clarification for a lay audience. Thus, it becomes increasingly important for the forensic psychiatrist to have expertise in many areas of psychiatry. However, the ethics of the American Academy of Psychiatry and the Law prohibit the expert witness from testifying in areas beyond his or her expertise. Training programs in forensic psychiatry have increased not only in number but also in the scope of the educational experiences of the fellows in training.

This book highlights the emerging issues in forensic psychiatry that every psychiatrist who enters the courtroom should be aware of before agreeing to become an expert witness. Even though the expert witness is often a consultant and does not testify, he or she still needs to know the issues surrounding the case.

The growth of forensic psychiatry has accelerated and the field will continue to expand and develop in the future. The expert psychiatrist needs to keep up with advances in the field as well as changes in the legal system. There are pitfalls and areas of concern that need to be avoided or clearly understood before entering the legal system. This book is essential for anyone willing to provide expert testimony and advice to lawyers and judges.

Robert L. Sadoff, M.D. is Clinical Professor of Forensic Psychiatry and Director, Forensic Psychiatry Fellowship Program, Perelman School of Medicine, University of Pennsylvania.

CONTRIBUTORS

Steven J. Berkowitz, MD
Associate Professor of Clinical
    Psychiatry and Director
The Penn Center for Youth and
    Family Trauma Response
University of Pennsylvania,
    Perelman School of Medicine
Adjunct Associate Professor
Yale University Child Study Center
    Department of Psychiatry

Octavio Choi, MD, PhD
Assistant Professor
Department of Psychiatry
Oregon Health and Science
    University

Julia Curcio-Alexander, PhD
Supervising Psychologist and
    Coordinator of Evaluation Services
Joseph J. Peters Institute
Philadelphia

Helen M. Farrell, MD
Forensic Psychiatrist and Instructor
Department of Psychiatry
Harvard Medical School
Psychiatrist
Beth Israel Deaconess Medical Center
Boston

Nicole Foubister, MD
Assistant Professor Child and
    Adolescent Psychiatry
Assistant Professor Psychiatry
New York University School of
    Medicine
NYU Child Study Center
Department of Child and
    Adolescent Psychiatry
NYU College of Arts & Science

Manish A. Fozdar, MD
Triangle Forensic Neuropsychiatry,
    PLLC
Consulting Assistant Professor
    of Psychiatry, Duke University
    Medical Center
Adjunct Associate Professor,
    Campbell University

**Jacqueline Block Goldstein,
MSW**
Associate Director and Child
    Forensic Interviewer
Philadelphia Children's Alliance

Samson Gurmu, MD
Forensic Psychiatrist
State of New Jersey Department of
    Human Services
Division of Mental Health and
    Addiction Services at the Ann
    Klein Forensic Center
West Trenton
New Jersey

Daniel D. Langleben, MD
Associate Professor of Psychiatry
    and Distinguished Research
    Fellow
Annenberg Public Policy Center
Perelman School of Medicine
University of Pennsylvania

John K. Northrop, MD, PhD
Clinical Associate
Department of Psychiatry
Perelman School of Medicine
University of Pennsylvania

Mark R. Pressman, PhD
Licensed Psychologist
Sleep Medicine Services
and
Clinical Professor
Lankenau Institute for Medical
    Research
The Lankenau Hospital
Wynnewood, PA
Clinical Professor of Medicine
Jefferson Medical College
Adjunct Professor of Law
Villanova University

Susan E. Rushing, MD, JD
Department of Psychiatry
Perelman School of Medicine
University of Pennsylvania

Frank K. Tedeschi, MD
Clinical Assistant Professor
Department of Child and
    Adolescent Psychiatry
New York University School of
    Medicine
and
Attending Psychiatrist
Department of Child and
    Adolescent Psychiatry
Bellevue Hospital, New York

Clarence Watson, JD, MD
Clinical Assistant Professor
Department of Psychiatry
Perelman School of Medicine
University of Pennsylvania

Kenneth J. Weiss, MD
Clinical Professor
Department of Psychiatry
Perelman School of Medicine
University of Pennsylvania

**Alexander R. N. Westphal,
    MD, PhD**
Assistant Professor
Department of Psychiatry
Yale School of Medicine

INTRODUCTION

BY KENNETH J. WEISS AND CLARENCE WATSON

The psychiatric expert witness: boon to jurisprudence or necessary evil? From our own perspective, we fly the banner of enlightening courts with science. To civil plaintiffs' attorneys, we can be the key to a big payoff; to their defense counterparts, we can be a means to keep purse strings tight. Prosecutors in criminal cases count on us to find no link between mental state and behavior, whereas defense attorneys trust that science will explain or even excuse deviance. Judges, meanwhile, run the gamut from cynical to adulatory. How the public regards us is often a matter of which sensational trial appears on television. More often than not, scientific witnesses, especially in mental health, are viewed as scripted performers in a "battle of the experts." Yet, psychiatry appears wedded to jurisprudence and we must make the best of it—or choose to observe from the sidelines. We trust that, by reading the contributions to this volume, clinicians will be better prepared to engage in medicolegal matters.

PSYCHIATRIC EXPERTISE: WHAT MAKES IT FORENSIC?

The word *forensic*, the adjective of the Latin *forum*, refers to matters in the public sphere, such as the market or court. Often conflated with the more famous forensic pathology, forensic psychiatry and psychology are not studies of death. They are *applications* of psychiatry and psychology, each having its own professional body of literature, training, and accreditation. Mental health professionals and other expert witnesses are visitors to an alien planet when they enter the legal arena. Those of us who specialize in forensic work can become comfortable with the language, procedures, and overall feeling of legal proceedings. Still, experts who are accustomed to being "captain of the ship" in their own domains may be jolted by differences between mental health treatment settings and litigation.

Implied in the word *forensic*, mental health applications to litigation (criminal or civil) are conducted in a public setting. In contrast to the sanctity of the therapeutic encounter, once a person's mental state is brought into legal proceedings, what was private is no longer so. Of course, there are limits, restrictions, and ethical constraints on certain disclosures. Nevertheless, raising mental health issues, especially in adversarial proceedings, can put intimate—even shameful—details of someone's life under a microscope. For this reason, it is not advisable for mental health professionals to blur roles by giving expert testimony for their own clients, a situation referred to as "wearing two hats."[1] The two-hats problem diminishes objectivity when testifying about one's patient and can have a disruptive effect on the therapeutic relationship.

EXPERT WITNESSES: HISTORICAL AND CULTURAL ASPECTS

Justice systems have used expert witnesses for centuries. In America, applied scientific knowledge emerged and accelerated through the 19th century. Perceiving that there was money to be made, attorneys and experts often abused the system by offering opinions that lacked scientific integrity. Although psychiatric matters were hardly the only application, since our subject matter was not immediately perceptible to the average person, psychiatric experts have often been the subject of suspicion if not outright scorn. Europeans understood experts as aids to justice. Accordingly, our counterparts may wonder what all the fuss is about—why our experts are exhaustively vetted and often kept on a short leash. Our understanding, in part, is based on the tension between science and the law, a subject too big and philosophical to cover here. The tension has to do with the differential rates of change between law (slow) and science (fast, and accelerating). Scientists, eager to apply knowledge to litigation, among other things, feel the need to drag legal proceedings into the current century, whereas legislatures and jurists act as gatekeepers, so that science does not lead the law. Our position, as seasoned professionals, is that both sides are right. It is not the purpose of this book to analyze jurisprudence or to influence legislatures as much as it is to help potential expert witnesses find the right combination of science and timing to ensure that what they say is in the interest of justice. Too little science makes us look out of step with other fields, whereas premature applications may be like lead balloons.

Trial attorneys cannot convey scientific evidence by themselves. Expert witnesses are required to educate judges and juries, who are considered laypersons in relation to the field of inquiry. It is not enough for a criminal defense lawyer, for example, to suggest to the jury that the manifestly disturbed defendant (at the defense table responding to hallucinations) could not have been sane at the time of a homicide. No, an expert witness must provide a diagnosis and "connect the dots" between this condition and the legal standard for criminal responsibility in that jurisdiction (there are differences from state to state). It would make sense that a court could appoint an expert to provide this indispensible function. History tells us, however, that there is great resistance from lawyers to dispense with partisan experts.

There was a huge spike in using forensic expertise in the 19th century, coupled with extensive treatises on forensic medicine, toxicology, and the jurisprudence of insanity.[2-4] The culture of American jurisprudence shifted toward misuse of experts, many of whom lacked credentials and personal integrity.[5] To a degree, the justice system has never fully recovered. Whenever there is a battle of the experts, citizens tend to look on it as more of a circus than a truth-seeking venture. One of this book's objectives is to push the tide the other way.

Tension is also found in the interplay between the ends of justice, the march of science, the manner in which experts interpret science, and trends in societal values. This is best illustrated in a succession of cases of the insanity defense in England[6] and in America. Before 1800, traditional jurisprudence was that mental excuses for behavior were to be reserved for those whose capacities were no keener than those of a wild beast. But in 1800, a deluded James Hadfield shot at King George of England and was acquitted. This thrust the "delusion test" for insanity into the forefront of jurisprudence, to the dismay of Parliament. The legislature quickly passed a law permitting the confinement of insanity acquittees, and Hadfield spent his remaining 40 years in institutions.

Then in 1840, it was Queen Victoria's turn to face a madman, when Edward Oxford attempted to assassinate her with pistols. Oxford was found insane and confined for decades. Three years later, a deluded Scotsman, Daniel M'Naghten, believing he was shooting Prime Minister Robert Peal, shot his secretary, Mr. Drummond. By then, defense attorney Cockburn took advantage of an American textbook, Isaac Ray's *A Treatise on the Medical Jurisprudence of Insanity*.[4] Indeed, M'Naghten was acquitted by reason of insanity, which created tension in Buckingham Palace and Parliament. The House of Lords quickly responded to restrict the use of the insanity defense, creating M'Naghten's Rules. The surviving rule, adopted by many states in America, is a purely "cognitive" test: Acquittal depends on a thought disorder causing a "defect of reason" such that, at the time of the act in question, the defendant did not know that the behavior was wrong. This narrow definition of insanity continues to be a problem for expert witnesses, who might want to introduce evidence of emotional or impulse-control disorders into a defense—and may even demonstrate the basis for them via neuroimaging.

In America, the insanity standard came into focus when John Hinckley shot President Reagan in 1981. At that time, the federal standard for insanity included both cognitive (appreciating wrongfulness) and volitional (reduced ability to conform one's behavior) prongs. Hinckley was acquitted in his 1982 trial, where an early use of psychiatric testimony based on brain computed tomography findings was permitted after a difficult process. More important, the public outrage at the acquittal, despite Hinckley's civil commitment, gave rise to the Insanity Defense Reform Act of 1984. This Act restricted the role of the expert witness and has been viewed as an aid to prosecutors. Meanwhile, there is no constitutionally mandated right to an insanity plea for criminal defendants and, as of 2012, the U.S. Supreme Court has declined to consider the matter.[7] Kansas, Montana, Idaho, and Utah have abolished insanity pleas, further restricting the possibility of expert witnesses shedding light on criminal behavior.

OPINING ON THE TRUTH: HOLY GRAIL OR THE FATE OF ICARUS?

Might it be possible to dispense with partisan experts in favor of neutral conveyors of scientific knowledge? Can scientists be trusted to say, for example, if a witness is lying? What about the credibility of a victim's assertions? These types of questions have vexed practitioners, courts, and legal scholars for many years. In practice, expert witnesses are not called to tell judges or juries the underlying truth of a matter (e.g., guilt or innocence, liability, or veracity). These are the ultimate issues, the exclusive province of fact finders (judges and juries). It should not be the goal of scientists to replace the jury system. Rather, we are expected to aid the fact finders by shedding light on matters that are beyond ordinary knowledge. While the notion that an expert witness can see the ultimate truth of a matter is seductive, it is not in keeping with legal procedures and rules of evidence, as Dr. Watson will review in the next chapter. When an expert witness gets too close to the province of the fact finder, the testimony may be fatally flawed and barred from the proceedings. Thus, what seemed to be a quest for the holy grail could turn out to be an exercise in flying too close to the sun. Like Icarus, the expert motivated by hubris will crash, and in doing so will damage the client.

Trial lawyers, criminal and civil, are often quick to import scientific knowledge and techniques in support of legal arguments. X-radiation, for example, was discovered by Roentgen in 1895 and applied to photography of interior anatomy. Within a year, a patient had sued a doctor for malpractice, arguing that the doctor had missed a leg fracture sustained in a fall, diagnosed as a soft-tissue injury. The Colorado case *Smith v. Grant* was the first in which X-ray images played a role in determining a standard-of-care question.[8] As it was, malpractice suits were on the rise in turn-of-the-century America. During the litigation, the court determined that, despite defense counsel's objection, photographs using the X-ray process could be produced as secondary evidence (only in conjunction with expert testimony), on a par with maps and charts. The matter was settled, but the issues raised about seeking deeper—or definitive—truth remain with us.[9,10] Several of our authors will discuss the problems and prospects for the use of indirect data in answering legal questions. The main thing to remember is that these emerging technologies do not stand on their own as evidence; they support the expert's opinions, which must be defended sometimes in pretrial evidentiary hearings.

In the 19th century, psychiatrists provided expert testimony on their observations of individuals. Rather than giving direct opinions on legal matters, they would respond to hypothetical ("what if") questions. There was little other science to shed light on questions of mental states. Phrenology, dominant through much of the 19th century, did not make its way into the courtroom by way of a psychiatric defense.[11] Yet, the search for indirect markers of psychological truth remained an elusive goal. The most famous example of this is the use of the polygraph as a means of lie detection. Other 20th-century techniques, such as hypnosis and narcosis (truth serum), have had their day but remain controversial because the results tend to border on the forbidden area of prejudicing the jury. Inferential data from the autonomic nervous system, such as from the polygraph, have a clinical truth but lack forensic power. The universal phenomenon of blushing may indicate many things; this is the subject of a recent book.[12] As legendary Harvard psychiatry professor Dr. Elvin Semrad used to say, "The autonomic nervous system doesn't lie." That may be true in the treatment context, where blushing or dry mouth betrays the patient's words. But we think that Dr. Semrad, who likely was never cross-examined, would agree that courts require a different type of truth, one that is usually beyond the reach of the testifying expert. Besides, as criminologist Adrian Raine points out, psychopaths lie with their autonomic nervous systems as well as through their mouths.[13] So much for clinical impressionism!

In the early 20th century, Harvard psychologist Hugo Münsterberg, intent on applying science to the courtroom, touted a scientific method for verifying eyewitness testimony.[14] After a series of psychology experiments using word-association analysis, he believed he had broken through the barrier between the laboratory and the real world, thus initiating forensic psychology. Professor Münsterberg, otherwise known for originating applied and forensic psychologies in America, was severely criticized, setting back the use of expert testimony in cases of questionable memory. The most severe criticism came from John H. Wigmore, dean of Northwestern Law School, whose name is virtually synonymous with the law of evidence. Around the same time, Swiss psychiatrist C. G. Jung researched a word-association test as a clinical shortcut to uncover neurotic complexes. Sigmund Freud, skeptical of Jung's methods, belittled his colleague while lecturing to a group of law students in Vienna in 1906.[15,16] Freud took a dim view of forensic applications of psychoanalytic theory and generally refused to participate in trials. He knew intuitively the difference between psychological theory and forensically robust testimony.

The idea of technologically aided truth finding will be echoed in this volume. First, Clarence Watson will review the standards for scientific certainty, including the *Frye*[17] test for general acceptance of scientific findings and the *Daubert*[18] test for admissibility. In the 1923 D.C. Circuit Court opinion in *U.S. v. Frye*, the proposed scientific lie detection (systolic blood pressure elevation) was rejected as evidence because it lacked acceptance within the scientific community. In Chapter 6, Octavio Choi will review the iterations of lie detection and the circumstances under which expert testimony can be admitted. The search for truth goes on, but will it be found in brain function or structure?

THE WORK PRODUCT

Expert witnesses rarely enter the courtroom, because more than 9 out of 10 cases, civil and criminal, do not result in trials. The reason is simple: Settlements are often a safer course than placing one's fate in the hands of strangers. On the civil side, a negotiated or arbitrated settlement means that the injured party, the plaintiff, will receive monetary damages in a smaller amount than hoped. The defendant, by settling, will have eliminated the possibility of a huge jury award. On the criminal side, a settled case means that the defendant has accepted responsibility for an unlawful act, but often one that carries a smaller sentence (e.g., for assault with a weapon rather than attempted murder). The settlement, when approved by the parties and the judge, ends the litigation and precludes a trial. This outcome, however, does not eliminate the role of expert witnesses. To the contrary: Experts may be crucial in bringing closure to these difficult situations.

If most cases are never tried, why would we bother to write about expert testimony? By *testimony* we are referring to the totality of the expert's work product. Some professionals serve as "consulting experts," who assist attorneys on the sidelines and never issue reports or testimony. Most professionals engaged by attorneys are "testifying experts," who form scientific opinions on matters before the court, put their findings into written reports, and provide live testimony under oath in depositions or trials.

By far the most prevalent type of work product is the written report. Indeed, more often than not, the expert report is the only work product in a case; its importance cannot be overestimated. The psychiatric expert report has been the standard since the 19th century and is the subject of a book of its own.[19] As Clarence Watson will explain in Chapter 1, most expert medical opinions, psychiatric or otherwise, must be expressed to a level of confidence called "reasonable medical certainty" (or a variant, such as reasonable scientific certainty or probability). Over the years, legal authorities have arrived at this convention, which, simply stated, says that experts must state that it is more likely than not that there is a causal relationship in the matter at hand—for example, that the motor vehicle accident caused traumatic stress, or that schizophrenia caused a cognitive defect that prevented someone from knowing that an otherwise criminal act was wrong. Sometimes this convention is called the 51% rule, although generally we would not use a quantitative description; it is just understood by the lawyers and judge. A higher threshold of certainty is required in civil commitment, where there is a potential for deprivation of liberty by virtue of what we say. By contrast, the expert witness' burden is never as high as that of a criminal juror, who, to vote for conviction of a defendant, must find that the prosecution proved its case beyond a reasonable doubt. Legal authorities recognize that scientific testimony cannot be held to that standard. Even fingerprint analysis[20] and polygraphic lie detection[21] are not infallible and can be challenged, but do not stand alone as proof.

It is clear that expert witnesses play a supporting role in trials, although sometimes that role is the center of attention. This is true in medical malpractice cases, where the parties and trier of fact look to experts to define whether the defendant clinician's actions were above or below an acceptable level of competence (standard of care). We will not be focusing on malpractice matters in this book. How, then, does the expert witness apply his or her education, specialized knowledge, skill, and experience to legal matters? Unlike the medical setting that asks us a health-related question, the legal setting always engages us with a legal question. We are rarely expected to answer the legal question itself—only to shed light on it so that a jury or judge can decide. Examples of typical legal questions are: Does an individual have the mental capacity to enter into a contract? Was an employee injured by the actions of the employer? Is a criminal defendant's mental illness a bar to participating in a trial? Although one can see how expert testimony would play a pivotal role in aiding the decision maker, the witness is always subservient to the court (judge) and its officers (attorneys). The fact that there are usually expert opinions on both sides of cases should keep us humble. However, it does not always prevent some experts from acting arrogant or grandiose, which can be harmful to the case and to the profession. And while many expert witnesses in adversarial settings identify with the cause of the party that hired them, assuming the role of combatant may reduce objectivity and scientific credibility.

ETHICS AND THE EXPERT WITNESS

The persuasive power of the expert witness must be used with caution and mindfulness. As Robert Sadoff has urged, the expert must try to be efficacious while minimizing harm.[22] Aware of the need for professional standards and the importance of maintaining credibility in non-healthcare settings, the professions of forensic psychiatry and forensic psychology have developed ethical guidelines.[23,24] Because the aim of this book is to familiarize forensic practitioners with emerging applications, we would be remiss if we did not review essential ethics. It is especially relevant to review ethics when we contemplate using scientific information that might be considered speculative. The expert witness must remember to stay a step back from any emotional attachment to a diagnostic tool or interviewing technique to ensure that the focus of the testimony is on the legal question and not on self-promotion. The following are key tenets of forensic psychiatric ethics, excerpted from the guidelines published by the American Academy of Psychiatry and the Law (AAPL).[23]

The AAPL ethics guidelines begin by acknowledging the complexity and role ambiguity created by physicians working within legal settings: "Psychiatrists in a forensic role are called upon to practice in a manner that balances competing duties to the individual and to society. In doing so, they should be bound by underlying ethical principles of respect for persons, honesty, justice, and social responsibility"."[23]

The fact of a shift in the forensic psychiatrist's role from healthcare provider to objective evaluator does not lessen or eliminate the need for confidentiality. While it may be true that placing one's mental state into litigation renders the information public to a degree, forensic professionals are bound to adhere to enhanced requirements for privacy and declaration of intent. Thus, the AAPL guidelines call for the following:[25]

- "Psychiatrists should maintain confidentiality to the extent possible, given the legal context."
- "Special attention should be paid to the evaluee's understanding of medical confidentiality."
- "A forensic evaluation requires notice to the evaluee and to collateral sources of reasonably anticipated limitations on confidentiality."
- "Information or reports derived from a forensic evaluation are subject to the rules of confidentiality that apply to the particular evaluation, and any disclosure should be restricted accordingly."

Practically speaking, the subject of the evaluation (or legally authorized representative) will need to know that there is no treatment relationship, that the information will be shared, and, if applicable, that the results of the assessment could be used by the adverse party in the litigation. The individual's consent should be obtained, except when the assessment has been court ordered. In that case, the subject should also be informed of the consequences of refusal to cooperate.

The AAPL guidelines call for honesty and striving for objectivity: "The adversarial nature of most legal processes presents special hazards for the practice of forensic psychiatry...Psychiatrists should not distort their opinion in the service of the retaining party."[25] Adherence to these principles requires self-awareness and vigilance. The main pitfalls are overidentification with the retaining attorney's legal position and the shading of one's position to earn more.[25] Basing financial compensation to the expert on the outcome of the case (contingency fee), for example, is forbidden. Another way to ensure objectivity is for the expert to conduct comprehensive evaluations: "Psychiatrists practicing in a forensic role enhance the honesty and objectivity of their work by basing their forensic opinions, forensic reports and forensic testimony on all available data."[25] Thus, the cherry-picking of data or the intentional disregard of information that could conflict with the referring attorney's goal lacks integrity. While it may be ethical for lawyers to do so (with the exception of criminal prosecutors), our code tells us otherwise.

As we discuss emerging applications of psychiatry to the law, the question may arise in the reader's mind as to whether to get involved in a case requiring knowledge outside of general psychiatry (e.g., polysomnography, brain development, or neuroimaging): "Expertise in the practice of forensic psychiatry should be claimed only in areas of actual knowledge, skills, training, and experience. When providing expert opinion, reports, and testimony, psychiatrists should present their qualifications accurately and precisely."[25] A treating psychiatrist may send a patient to a diagnostic radiologist for brain imaging and use the reading to guide therapy. A more confident clinician will also read the images. However, when it comes to using meaningful interpretations of images to answer legal questions, the clinician as expert witness must either be prepared to explain thoroughly the science and technology behind the imaging technique or to delegate it to a neuroradiologist. In terms of representing one's credentials, the radiologist will not pretend to give a behavioral analysis of the findings and the psychiatrist will not overclaim expertise on technical matters. The AAPL guidelines add that "there are areas of special expertise, such as the evaluation of children, persons of foreign cultures, or prisoners, that may require special training or expertise."[25] Thus, as you explore the potential applications in this book, bear in mind that testimony must be backed up by technical knowledge or specialized experience that will hold up to cross-examination.

EMERGING APPLICATIONS: A PREVIEW

Our theme is integration of mental health expertise into civil and criminal proceedings. Each chapter can stand alone as a review of a type of litigation requiring expert testimony. We encourage all readers to read Chapter 1 first, to be grounded in the rules of the game. Beyond that, readers can explore the applications as need or interest arises. We have incorporated *DSM-5* nomenclature into these discussions, since finding a common clinical language is often a key to formulating and communicating forensic opinions. Throughout the book we have avoided a prescriptive approach, understanding that each practitioner will incorporate current practice and case law into reasonably evidence-based reports and testimony. We urge all practitioners to consult local statutes and court opinions in preparation of their work product, as the examples given here may not be applicable in all jurisdictions.

In Chapter 1, Clarence Watson will discuss the rules governing expert testimony: when experts are used, what their qualifications must be, and, to a degree, what they can say. It is important to remember that these rules (e.g., the Federal Rules of Evidence) were invented by lawyers in the interest of justice. That is, we experts do not make the rules—but we must conform to them. You may indeed be the world's expert in a scientific matter, but your opinions on a legal matter may be rejected. How is this possible? As Dr. Watson explains, the rules governing expert witnesses tell us that testimony must be helpful to the "trier of fact" (jury or judge) without prejudicing the outcome—in addition to being scientifically sound. The importance of this principle, for the purposes of this book, cannot be overemphasized. Our contributors will be discussing applications of psychiatric testimony that may be challenged as, for example, too prejudicial or ahead of their time in terms of scientific weight.

We continue the specific content areas with chapters that include two broad categories: human developmental perspectives in illuminating legal issues (Chapters 2 through 5) and technological advances that support expert testimony in emerging fields of interest (Chapters 6 through 10). In Chapter 2, Nicole Foubister and Frank Tedeschi discuss how knowledge of human psychological development informs testimony about children and adolescents. This is increasingly important, as the distinctions between the juvenile and adult brain structure and functioning are played out in courtrooms and legislatures. In Chapter 3, Julia Curcio-Alexander, Jacqueline Block Goldstein, and Kenneth Weiss explore child sexual abuse by way of interpreting victims' behavior. They note the phenomenon of "accommodation" of the victim, which can lead to difficulty prosecuting the perpetrator. The question they discuss is how clinical evidence of accommodation (such as denial or recantation) can be expressed in court without the testimony being considered incriminating against the defendant. In Chapter 4, John Northrop and Steven Berkowitz add the special circumstances of adverse childhood experiences and early trauma to the discussion of brain development as it pertains to morality, impulse control, and accountability. While it may sound like a cliché to associate a deprived childhood with later antisocial behavior, we now have science to back it up. The authors take the position that adverse childhood experiences are, in fact, brain injuries. They also empha-size that labels, such as posttraumatic stress disorder, are often insufficient to describe the downstream effects of maltreatment, as manifestations may take multiple forms. Translating that for juries may make big differences in outcomes, when culpability is in question. In Chapter 5, Kenneth Weiss and Alexander Westphal assess our knowledge of autism spectrum disorder as it applies to analysis of criminal responsibility. The apparent lack of empa-thy in autism spectrum disorder is a defect in Theory of Mind, distinguished from the callousness in psychopathy. The authors emphasize the importance of making this distinction for judges and juries.

Turning to more technology-based applications, we begin with Octavio Choi's discussion of neuroimaging and lie detection in Chapter 6. The question has now become: To what degree can expert witnesses speak to juries with-out invading their territory of truth finding? This is a deep and leading-edge subject that forces us to focus on the borders of science and behavior. The science behind lie detection has evolved since the era of word-association and systolic blood pressure tests. Here, Dr. Choi focuses on functional MRI imaging and takes us to the current limits of knowledge and legal admis-sibility. Clarence Watson, Mark Pressman, and Kenneth Weiss in Chapter 7 discuss scientific knowledge about parasomnias as they apply to analyses of criminal responsibility. How we measure consciousness and the capacity for criminal intent may be affected by disorders of sleep. While the law tells us that sleeping persons are incapable of committing crimes, the proof of sleep has become an intriguing challenge. In Chapter 8, Susan Rushing and Daniel Langleben explain how brain imaging can increase insight into human behavior in criminal and civil cases. The resulting testimony must conform to the rules of evidence and must not be substituted for ordinary clinical analysis. Increasingly, courts have been interested in measurable param-eters of brain development that inform sentencing and how culpability is decided. In Chapter 9, Manish Fozdar and Helen Farrell raise forensic issues in an especially active area of clinical concern: chronic traumatic encepha-lopathy. This condition may give rise to criminal and civil litigation and has become a fertile area for expert witnesses. Of special interest is the relation-ship between sports-induced chronic traumatic encephalopathy and claims that team owners, football helmet makers, and sports leagues share liability for possible dementia-related outcomes. Samson Gurmu and Kenneth Weiss take on the emerging interface of designer drugs and criminal responsibility in Chapter 10. Although there is little guidance from case law, the authors outline the potential avenues criminal defendants might take to diminish criminal responsibility. There is no civil right to present a defense of intoxi-cation, but when someone uses new substances with unknown effects, can a claim be made for involuntary intoxication? Here, as in other chapters, the authors will discuss types of testimony from both sides of the case.

Whereas the rules of evidence are not the domain of science, expert witnesses have responsibilities to maintain scientific integrity and to help triers of fact with their difficult jobs. There are many ways to assist legal processes, and each witness will develop a style that is ethical and informative. Accordingly, we have embraced an approach that explores each subject without being prescriptive or formulaic. We urge readers to use the information within these chapters as a launching point for fashioning reports and testimony, not necessarily as a blueprint for constructing the work product. It is our wish and that of the contributors to assist the justice system by demonstrating scientific progress while maintaining respect for legal traditions.

REFERENCES

1. Strasberger LH, Gutheil TG, Brodsky A. On wearing two hats: role conflict in serving as both psychotherapist and expert witness. *Am J Psychiatry.* 1997; 154(4): 448–456.
2. Beck TR. *Elements of Medical Jurisprudence.* Albany, NY: Webster & Skinners; 1823.
3. Wharton F, Stillé M. *A Treatise on Medical Jurisprudence.* Philadelphia, PA: Kay & Brother; 1855.
4. Ray I. *A Treatise on the Medical Jurisprudence of Insanity.* Boston, MA: Chas. Little & Jas. Brown; 1838.
5. Mohr JC. *Doctors and the Law: Medical Jurisprudence in Nineteenth-Century America.* Baltimore, MD: The Johns Hopkins University Press; 1993.
6. Eigen JP. *Witnessing Insanity: Madness and Mad-Doctors in the English Court.* New Haven, CT: Yale University Press; 1995.
7. Morse SJ, Bonnie RJ. Abolition of the insanity defense violates due process. *J Am Acad Psychiatry Law.* 2013; 41(4): 488–495.
8. Goldberg DS. The transformative power of X-rays in U.S. scientific & medical litigation: mechanical objectivity in *Smith v. Grant* (1896). *Perspect Science.* 2013; 21(1): 23–57.
9. Golan T. *Laws of Men and Laws of Nature: The History of Scientific Expert Testimony in England and America.* Cambridge, MA: Harvard University Press; 2004.
10. Weiss KJ. Head, examined: Clarence Darrow's X-ray vision of criminal responsibility. *J Psychiatry Law.* 2011; 39: 627–661.
11. Weiss KJ. Isaac Ray at 200: phrenology and expert testimony. *J Am Acad Psychiatry Law.* 2007; 35(3): 339–345.
12. Crozier WR, de Jong PJ, eds. *The Psychological Significance of the Blush.* New York: Cambridge University Press; 2013.
13. Raine A. *The Anatomy of Violence.* New York: Random House; 2013.
14. Münsterberg H. *On the Witness Stand: Essays on Psychology and Crime.* New York: Doubleday, Page & Co.; 1909.
15. Freud S: Psycho-analysis and the establishment of the facts in legal proceedings (1906). *The Standard Edition of the Complete Psychological Works of Sigmund Freud,* vol. 9. Edited and translated by J. Strachey. London: The Hogarth Press; 1959: 103–114 (editor's notes, pp. 99–102).

16. Weiss KJ. Classics in psychiatry and the law: Francis Wharton on involuntary confessions. *J Am Acad Psychiatry Law* 2012; 40: 67–80.
17. *Frye v. U.S.* 293 F. 1013 (D.C. Cir. 1923).
18. *Daubert v. Merrell Dow Pharmaceuticals, Inc.* 509 U.S. 579, 113 (1992).
19. Buchanan A, Norko MA. *The Psychiatric Report: Principles and Practice of Forensic Writing.* Cambridge, UK: Cambridge University Press; 2011.
20. Saks MJ. The legal and scientific evaluation of forensic science (especially fingerprint expert testimony). *Seton Hall Law Review.* 2003; 33(4): 1167–1187.
21. Grubin D. The polygraph and forensic psychiatry. *J Am Acad Psychiatry Law.* 2010; 38(4): 446–451.
22. Sadoff RL. *Ethical Issues in Forensic Psychiatry: Minimizing Harm.* Chichester, UK: John Wiley & Sons, Ltd; 2011.
23. American Academy of Psychiatry and the Law. Ethics guidelines for the practice of forensic psychiatry, adopted May 2005. Available online at www.aapl.org/ethics.htm. These guidelines are supplemental to the American Psychiatric Association's annotations to the American Medical Association's general ethics.
24. American Psychological Association. Specialty guidelines for forensic psychology. *Am Psychol.* 2013; 68(1): 7–19.
25. Mnookin JL. Expert evidence, partisanship, and epistemic competence. *Brooklyn Law Review.* 2008; 73(3): 1009–1033.

CHAPTER 1

Expert Testimony: Legal Principles

CLARENCE WATSON

" [T]he Law of Evidence] constitutes a most important part of human opinion; it has fluctuated with the vicissitudes of society; it has advanced with its progress, and declined with its degradation. For it was when all the resources of superstition were exhausted, when the relics which were the most awful of all guarantees in a barbarous age, failed to ensure the veracity of a witness, that the judge in mere despair and conscious of his inability to discover the truth, called upon Providence to supply by a special interposition, the want of human judgment, and sagacity" (pp. 2–3).[1] Through those words, Phillmore spoke to the necessary progress that had been made, even in his day, from an era of trials by ordeal and combat to the embrace of ancient Roman principles aimed at truth seeking amid contentious legal dispute.[1] *Ei incumbit probatio qui dicit, non qui negat*—the burden of the proof lies upon him who affirms, not he who denies—is one such ancient Roman tenet and represents a core legal principle that roots contemporary laws of evidence.

The law of evidence in the United States, as it is recognized today, represents a body of principles forged gradually over the centuries as citizens sought equitable resolution of legal disputes by the respective tribunals of their day. Infused with ancient Roman and medieval Norman ideals, English law was transported across the Atlantic along with the cultural customs of the British colonists in North America, and formed the foundation of the legal system in the United States.[2] Surprisingly, although humankind's legal tradition can be traced back to ancient roots, the law of evidence, as we know it today, was essentially nonexistent until the 18th century and, as such, is in its infancy by comparison.[3] Even at its beginnings, the focus of evidence law centered on the authentication of documents or *proof of writings*, while issues regarding oral testimony of witnesses received little to no attention, except for barring testimony from individuals with interests in the matter's outcome (including the disputing parties).[3] Naturally, rules related to expert scientific testimony during trials were absent, allowing experts to testify with virtual free rein and with little distinction from lay witnesses, who were also permitted to offer opinion testimony.[4]

Over the course of centuries, it has been well recognized and accepted that courts need expert testimony to deal with matters that lie outside of the experience of the judge and jury. However, over that same timeframe, a growing and palpable tension developed in the courtroom regarding the proper balance of the necessity of expert testimony against its potentially prejudicial effects. As Judge Learned Hand wrote in 1901: "No one will deny that the law should in some way effectively use expert knowledge wherever it will aid in settling disputes. The only question is as to how it can do so best" (p. 40).[5] This chapter traces the historical roots of the legal principles and rules of admissibility governing expert witness testimony in the United States. With the seminal 1923 D.C. Circuit Court decision of *Frye v. U.S.*[6] as our fulcrum point, we will explore the historical treatment of the expert witness and discuss contemporary legal principles regarding expert testimony.

EXPERT TESTIMONY BEFORE *FRYE*

The historical record reflects the longstanding participation of experts assisting in legal disputes over the centuries, although the nature of that participation has evolved over time. Prior to the more familiar practice of partisan experts in the courtroom, the use of expert knowledge by early British tribunals occurred in two forms: the special jury and expert advisors summoned by the court.[7] Members of the special jury were expressly selected for their special knowledge or expertise, as they were considered especially qualified to decide the merits of particular legal claims. Depending on the case, these juries of experts ranged from panels of cooks and fishmongers to all-female juries determining claims of pregnancy.[8] For example, in a 1351 case, a defendant, charged with selling rotten food, faced a jury of cooks and fishmongers, who decided the validity of the charges.[7] The practice of impaneling a jury of matrons *de ventre inspiciendo* to render a verdict of whether a woman was "quick with child" has been traced back to at least the 13th century.[8] Courts also summoned expert advisors to assist in cases where its knowledge was inadequate. For example, in a 1345 case involving an appeal of mayhem, a London court summoned surgeons to assist in determining whether a wound was fresh.[5] While these practices involved the use of experts in deciding legal matters, the expert did not yet provide direct testimony to a jury for the purpose of assisting it to render a verdict.

In 1901, Judge Learned Hand recounted some of the earliest recorded cases where expert testimony was submitted to the jury for its deliberation: *Alsop v. Bowtrell* (1620), *Rex v. Pembroke* (1678), and the Spencer Cowper case (1699).[5] In *Alsop v. Bowtrell*, a jury, deciding the legitimacy of a child, heard testimony from physicians that it was possible for a woman to deliver a child 40 weeks and 9 days after her husband's death. In the murder trial *Rex v. Pembroke*, physicians testified on behalf of the prosecution and the defense regarding the victim's cause of death and whether a man could die of wounds without fever. In the 1699 Spencer Cowper case, surgeons and sailors, who had been in sea fights, testified about whether the deceased had been drowned and whether a drowned body full of water would sink.

The use of expert testimony in this manner became more prevalent in the 18th century and thereafter, although the presence of evidentiary rules governing the admissibility of such testimony lagged significantly. In fact, there appeared to be only one legal criterion at that time for expert testimony: Individuals were qualified to speak as experts if they possessed special training or experience in the subject in question.[4] Of course, such a broad standard only dealt with the issue of relevance and did nothing to address the validity or reliability of the expert's testimony.

The English legal system's Adversarial Revolution in the 18th century and its associated rise of the partisan expert in the courtroom impelled the development of rules governing expert evidence.[4] Interestingly, prior to the 18th century, judges dominated criminal trials and lawyers were generally excluded from criminal proceedings. By the 1730s, judges began to assume a more neutral role and defense lawyers began to participate regularly in criminal trials, hence the Adversarial Revolution. As lawyers expanded their control over directing criminal defenses, two natural ramifications were the partisan selection of experts and explicit challenges to the admissibility of evidence. From those evidentiary challenges sprang two major legal doctrines: the hearsay doctrine and the opinion doctrine. These doctrines, for the first time, created a brighter boundary between the lay witness, who was no longer permitted to offer hearsay or opinion evidence, and the expert witness, who enjoyed a special exception to those rules.[4]

Lord Mansfield's 1782 opinion in the civil case of *Folkes v. Chadd*[9] hardened the acceptance of partisan experts to assist the jury and heralded the need for rules of evidence governing expert testimony.[10] In that case, plaintiffs claimed that the erection of a bank to prevent flooding caused the decay of a nearby harbor. Plaintiffs presented to the jury testimony by "[p]ilots, mariners, and other seamen" and an engineer to support their claims.[4] However, the trial judge excluded the testimony of the defendants' expert on the basis that his explanations were essentially opinions and could not be used by the jury to reach a verdict. On appeal, Lord Mansfield, Chief Justice of the Royal Court of King's Bench, found that the trial court erred in excluding the defense expert's testimony and held that opinion evidence by the defense expert was admissible. In clarifying the issue, Lord Mansfield reasoned, "…for in matters of science the reasonings of men of science can only be answered by men of science…In matters of science no other witnesses can be called…I cannot believe that where the question is, whether a defect arises from a natural or artificial cause, the opinions of men of science are not to be received…."[9]

Lord Mansfield's 1782 ruling appeared to be a resounding endorsement of expert testimony in the courtroom. However, as the use of expert witnesses became more commonplace during the 19th century, a swell of discontent with the practice could not be ignored, as U.S. legal scholars lamented the "evils" of expert testimony.[11] In 1909, Clearwater outlined some of those evils as follows: There are no satisfactory standards of expertness, and thus the testimony of charlatans is invited; the character of the evidence often given by so-called experts is partisan and unreliable; contradictory testimony of experts of apparently equal standing, having the same opportunities for acquiring knowledge of the facts, has a confusing effect upon juries; unprincipled self-styled experts are sometimes unscrupulously hired to support causes by specious and untruthful testimony; the litigant who has the longest purse can produce the most imposing array of experts; and the Bench sometimes permits the Bar to treat the accomplished and modest expert with studied contempt.[12]

In the early 20th century, there were widespread calls for reformative action against unbridled expert testimony in the courtroom. A common sentiment echoed throughout the legal system that unwary juries needed protection from misleading and corrupt expert testimony. Some U.S. jurisdictions responded by proposing or enacting legislation meant to leash expert testimony in American courts. In 1909, Michigan and Rhode Island had such legislation in place, while Maine was in the process of proposing similar laws.[13] However, this reformative approach through legislation proved unsuccessful, as these laws were eventually considered unconstitutional. It became clear that any clarity regarding the admissibility of expert testimony would only come from the courts through case law. A hint of clarity came in 1923 with the federal circuit court decision in *Frye v. United States*.[6]

Frye v. U.S.

In August 1921, James Alphonso Frye was arrested and charged with robbery in Washington, DC. During a police interrogation, Frye confessed to the unsolved murder of a prominent Washington, DC, physician in November 1920. Frye was then indicted for premeditated murder; however, prior to his trial in July 1922, Frye recanted his confession.[14] In an effort to determine the veracity of Frye's false confession claims, Dr. William Marston examined Frye using a systolic blood pressure deception test. Dr. Marston concluded that the test results indicated that Frye's claims of innocence were truthful and, consequently, Frye's defense proffered Dr. Marston's testimony regarding his findings.

However, the trial judge excluded Dr. Marston's testimony as inadmissible, and Frye was convicted of second-degree murder after a four-day trial. Frye immediately appealed his conviction, arguing that the trial court erred by refusing to allow Dr. Marston's testimony. The appellate court affirmed the lower court's decision and upheld Frye's conviction. The court found that Dr. Marston's deception test had not yet gained sufficient scientific validation to justify expert testimony regarding the test. The appellate court's opinion set out the *Frye* "general acceptance" standard regarding the admissibility of scientific evidence as follows:

> Just when a scientific principle or discovery crosses the line between the experimental and demonstrable stages is difficult to define. Somewhere in this twilight zone the evidential force of the principle must be recognized, and while courts will go a long way in admitting expert testimony deduced from a well-recognized scientific principle or discovery, the thing from which the deduction is made must be sufficiently established to have gained general acceptance in the particular field in which it belongs (p. 1014).[6]

The *Frye* standard required judges to determine two issues prior to admitting scientific evidence: (1) To what field did the proffered scientific principle belong? (2) Was the scientific principle generally accepted in that particular field? Although the *Frye* standard represented a major shift in courts' deliberations regarding scientific evidence, it was not without its critics. Criticisms of the *Frye* standard included concerns that many scientific principles did not fit neatly into a particular academic or professional field; that the threshold for "general acceptance" in a particular field was unclear; and that it was not clear whether the underlying scientific principle or the application of the scientific principle required general acceptance.[15]

Moreover, questions arose about whether *Frye*'s "general acceptance" test would erroneously exclude novel but otherwise reliable scientific principles that were too new to gain general acceptance in its field.[16] Despite these criticisms, the *Frye* test eventually became the gold standard in federal and state courts for the admissibility of scientific expert testimony over the next 50 years. The lure of a seemingly definitive method of ensuring the reliability of scientific evidence in the courtroom seemed irresistible.

U.S. FEDERAL RULES OF EVIDENCE OF 1975

While the *Frye* case appeared to provide much-needed clarity regarding the admissibility of scientific evidence, the body of evidence law as a whole remained in a state of disarray. Legal scholars proposing reformation of U.S. evidence law pointed to frequent inconsistencies in its application.[17] As Ladd argued, "A review of the history of evidence, with its spotted and often accidental growth, is persuasive proof of the need of introspective study of the law of evidence with a view to far-reaching improvement" (p. 218).[18]

In 1975, Congress responded by enacting the Federal Rules of Evidence, a codified set of rules that federal judges were required to apply in evidentiary matters. Despite Congress's intent to provide clarity, the Rules inadvertently contributed to the long-chronicled quandary regarding the admissibility of expert testimony. Specifically, the 1975 Federal Rule of Evidence (FRE) 702 addressed admissible expert testimony as follows:

> If scientific, technical, or other specialized knowledge will assist the trier of fact to understand the evidence or to determine a fact in issue, a witness qualified as an expert by knowledge, skill, experience, training, or education, may testify thereto in the form of opinion or otherwise.[19]

Patently absent from the language of FRE 702 was the *Frye* "general acceptance" test. Furthermore, it was unclear whether the *Frye* standard had even been considered, since no such indication appeared in the Advisory Committee Notes to Congress or during Congressional floor debates regarding the proposed Rules.[20] Naturally, the resulting uncertainty about whether *Frye's* "general acceptance" standard survived the adoption of the Rules threw courts into a tailspin.

Most state courts and some federal courts continued to follow the "general acceptance" standard, reasoning that the Rules did not explicitly abandon the established common law rule.[21] Other courts viewed the "general acceptance" standard as inconsistent with and implicitly rejected by FRE 402, which stated that "[a]ll relevant evidence is admissible, except as otherwise provided by the Constitution of the United States, by Act of Congress, by these rules, or by other rules prescribed by the Supreme Court pursuant to statutory authority."[22] Since the Rules did not include criteria regarding general acceptance in a scientific field to establish relevance, those courts viewed *Frye* as being implicitly repealed by the Rules.

The debate regarding the appropriate standard for admissibility of scientific evidence escalated throughout the 1980s and early 1990s. Growing concerns about "junk science" or unreliable scientific testimony in the courtroom fueled the debate.[23] The perception that the law extended "equal dignity to the opinions of charlatans and Nobel Prize winners" with only lay juries to make the distinction was unsettling to legal scholars.[24] Ultimately, the U.S. Supreme Court weighed in on the debate and clarified the status of the *Frye* "general acceptance" standard in the face of FRE 702 with its 1993 ruling in *Daubert v. Merrell Dow Pharmaceuticals.*[25]

Daubert v. Merrell Dow Pharmaceuticals

In 1993, the U.S. Supreme Court answered the question debated by the legal community since the Federal Rules of Evidence were enacted in 1975: Did the *Frye* "general acceptance" standard survive FRE 702? The Court's answer was outlined in its opinion in *Daubert v. Merrell Dow Pharmaceuticals.*[25] In *Daubert*, two child plaintiffs sued Merrell Dow, alleging that their mothers' ingestion during pregnancy of Merrell Dow's antiemetic product, Bendectin, caused their birth defects. The district court granted Merrell Dow's motion for summary judgment upon consideration of an affidavit by defendant's expert that epidemiological studies had not established a statistically significant association between birth defects and Bendectin. The district court rejected plaintiffs' expert testimony that test tube and animal studies demonstrated a link between the drug and birth defects because, in the court's view, that evidence was not generally accepted in its field. The Ninth Circuit Court of Appeals affirmed the district court's decision.

On certiorari, the U.S. Supreme Court vacated the lower court's decision, holding that the Federal Rules of Evidence superseded *Frye*'s "general acceptance" test. The Court's opinion designated the judge—not the scientific community—as the gatekeeper in determining whether relevant scientific evidence met the reliability threshold necessary to be admissible. To assist judges with this determination, the court offered nonexclusive factors that may be considered when deciding the admissibility of scientific evidence: (1) whether the theory or technique in question can be and has been tested, (2) whether the theory or technique has been subject to peer review and publication, (3) whether the theory or technique has a known or potential rate of error, (4) whether standards exist for control of the theory's or technique's operation, and (5) whether the theory or technique has attracted widespread acceptance within a relevant scientific community. Interestingly, the Court included acceptance in the relevant scientific community as a factor to consider, despite setting aside the *Frye* test. In the Court's view, a scientific community's "general acceptance" is only one of many factors that should be considered in admissibility determinations.

While *Daubert* clarified the status of the *Frye* standard, it left open other issues regarding the admissibility of expert testimony, which were later addressed by the Court. In *General Electric Co. v. Joiner*,[26] the Supreme Court reaffirmed the judge's gatekeeper role and ruled that the appropriate review standard for a judge's decision to exclude expert evidence is the abuse of discretion standard. The *Joiner* decision also highlighted the gatekeeper's authority to scrutinize the connectivity between an expert's proffered opinion and the data used to support that opinion. In *Kumho Tire Co., Ltd. v. Carmichael*,[27] the Supreme Court addressed the issue of whether the *Daubert* ruling only applied to expert testimony based on scientific principles rather than testimony based on skill and experience-based knowledge. The Court held that *Daubert* criteria were to be applied by the judges in a flexible and nonexhaustive manner to ensure the reliability of not only scientific principle-based evidence, but *all* relevant expert evidence. Accordingly, testimony in nonlaboratory-based sciences, or "soft sciences," such as psychology, sociology, and economics, appropriately fall within the judge's gatekeeper scrutiny, as outlined in *Daubert*, to ensure its reliability in the courtroom.

While *Daubert* and its progeny resolved critical issues regarding admissibility standards for expert testimony in federal courts, not all state jurisdictions follow the federal rules or the *Daubert* decision. In fact, while some states have embraced the *Daubert* ruling, other state jurisdictions have explicitly rejected *Daubert* in favor of the *Frye* standard.[28] As a result, the *Frye* test remains the prevailing standard in some states, and expert testimony in those jurisdictions must satisfy the "general acceptance" requirement before being presented to a jury. Therefore, it is important for testifying experts to be aware of the jurisdiction's applicable admissibility standard by which their testimony will be measured and challenged. The purpose of these standards is to ensure that an expert's opinions are sound and reliable, and not mere speculation.

EXPERTS IN THE COURTROOM

Long before the applicable admissibility standard issue is raised in the courtroom, attorneys wrestling with the decision to proffer scientific testimony must consider a crucial question: Will expert testimony be *helpful* to the fact finder in deciding a particular case? This question reflects the requirement that expert testimony must assist the judge or jury in deciding a factual issue that falls outside of ordinary knowledge or experience. Of course, to be helpful to the jury, the content of the expert's proffered testimony must be relevant to some issue in the case. Expert testimony deemed irrelevant, and therefore *unhelpful*, will be excluded as a matter of law.

A judge may also exclude expert testimony on matters commonly known or experienced by the average layperson, since that testimony can be considered unhelpful and potentially prejudicial. The exclusion of such testimony can be justified by concerns that experts are able to "assume a posture of mystic infallibility in the eyes of a jury of laymen" and could unduly influence or mislead jurors on issues that they are already equipped to consider.[29] There are times, however, where experts may be permitted to testify about matters within the average layperson's knowledge or experience. In situations where an expert's professional training or experience can provide a more in-depth understanding of matters commonly known or experienced by average jurors, such testimony may be considered helpful and properly admitted to a jury.

While expert testimony must be helpful and assist the fact finder, it cannot overreach into the province of the jury with opinions regarding witness credibility or determinations of the criminal or civil liability of involved parties.[30] The job of the testifying expert is to offer specialized knowledge where it is needed in order to *assist* the jury in effectively performing its exclusive function: reaching just verdicts based on the evidence. It is the role of the expert to educate the jury, not replace it. It is role of the jury to weigh witness credibility and decide the ultimate issue—the verdict. Courts will generally allow experts to offer opinions that embrace the ultimate issue, while juries are empowered to assign weight to such opinions against all of the evidence presented in a case.

To be helpful to the fact finder, an expert must be qualified to discuss the subject about which the expert testimony is being offered. The reasoning for this rule is plain: The purpose of expert testimony is to assist the jury in drawing its inferences regarding factual issues more reliably than it would unaided. Expert testimony by individuals who are not qualified in the subject matter to which they are testifying cannot fulfill this purpose. Accordingly, the trial judge must determine whether a proffered expert possesses the requisite specialized knowledge regarding particular factual issues that jurors will consider in reaching a verdict.

The presence or absence of academic credentials does not necessarily determine whether a witness will qualify as an expert. In some situations, experience alone may suffice, as long as the expert's experience affords a degree of expertise analogous to that of formally educated experts. The type of qualifications required by a court will depend on the nature of the opinions being offered by the expert. Hence, an expert's qualifications may be based on formal or informal education, experience, or a combination of these factors, depending on the proffered testimony. A judicial determination of a proffered expert's knowledge, training, experience, and education will take place in light of the specific opinion in question.

In fields such as medicine, which have become increasingly technical and specialized, experts must take special care only to offer opinions within their scope of expertise; otherwise, they run the risk of having their testimony excluded. For example, it is well accepted that being a physician alone does not qualify one to offer an opinion in every type of medical malpractice case. Similarly, not every mental health professional will necessarily be qualified as an expert to testify to every mental health question presented in court.

Even when an expert is qualified to offer testimony that is relevant to a legal matter, a judge has the discretion to exclude such testimony, if its prejudicial effect outweighs its probative value. Expert testimony that is relevant but nonetheless likely to mislead or confuse the jury may be barred as unduly prejudicial. For example, an appellate court upheld a district court's decision to exclude a psychologist's testimony regarding the reliability of eyewitness identifications on the basis that the testimony would likely confuse or mislead the jury.[31] In that case, the defendant attempted to appeal his robbery convictions, alleging that the district court erred in excluding his expert's testimony about factors that have an adverse impact on eyewitness identifications.

Given the potential pitfalls that experts may face when offering opinions in the courtroom, it is important for the expert to be aware of admissibility requirements in the relevant jurisdiction. Consultation with the retaining attorney to ensure that the expert's report and opinion satisfy the applicable admissibility standard is a prudent step. Experts should refrain from offering opinions that lie outside of their scope of expertise in order to preserve their role as a reliable educator in the courtroom.

REASONABLE MEDICAL CERTAINTY

When psychiatrists and other physicians provide expert opinions to the court through reports or testimony, they are often asked by attorneys to state their opinions with "reasonable medical certainty" or "reasonable medical probability." Similarly, nonphysician experts may be asked to state their opinions with "reasonable scientific certainty." While these phrases have become part of the standard lexicon in cases where medical or scientific expert testimony is introduced, there has been confusion among attorneys, judges, and experts about the precise meaning of those phrases.[32,33]

Moreover, the obscure and mysterious origin of these phrases has been noted in the legal literature, adding to the haze surrounding their use.[34] Lewin traces the genesis of "reasonable medical certainty" to the early 20th century and the Illinois Bar's attempt to reconcile the troublesome application of two evidentiary rules adopted by the Illinois Supreme Court: the "reasonable-certainty rule" and the "ultimate-issue rule."[33] The reasonable-certainty rule excluded testimony about future damages that were not reasonably certain to be incurred; the ultimate-issue rule prohibited expert witnesses from expressing definitive opinions regarding ultimate issues reserved for the jury, such as causation. Accordingly, medical experts in personal injury matters were required to testify with reasonable certainty about future damages but were banned from giving definitive opinions concerning causation. Lewin[33] argued that plaintiffs' attorneys, seeking to avoid the tripwire set by these rules, devised the "reasonable medical certainty" language to elicit favorable expert testimony safely. Between the 1930s and 1960s, the phrase "reasonable medical certainty" became firmly embedded within legal parlance nationwide.

Regardless of its origin, the precise meaning of "reasonable medical certainty" eluded the very experts from whom those words were expected to emanate. Rappeport[32] pointed out that some physicians believed that the phrase was equivalent to "beyond a reasonable doubt," while others viewed it as meaning a "preponderance of the evidence." Diamond argued that the phrase should represent "the psychiatrist's highest level of confidence in the validity and reliability of his opinion," which is based on clinical judgment and is not translatable into the legal standards of proof used by juries during deliberations.[35]

As it currently stands, "reasonable medical certainty" means that a physician believes his or her opinion to be "more likely than not" true or accurate. The phrase communicates to jurors the degree of clinical confidence that an expert assigns to an opinion, which was reached by the application of specialized knowledge to the facts of the case. It is usually insufficient to couch expert opinion in terms of "possibility." Failure to express opinions with the requisite level of certainty or probability (depending on the jurisdiction's preference) may be detrimental to the case of the expert's retaining attorney. Accordingly, the prudent expert should be aware of the level of certainty required by the jurisdiction in which he or she is testifying. Before offering an opinion in an unfamiliar jurisdiction, the expert is advised to consult with the retaining attorney regarding any nuanced but mandatory jurisdictional language, such as "reasonable medical probability," "reasonable psychiatric certainty," or any other variant.

CONCLUSION

The role of the expert witness is to educate the court on matters that lie beyond the sphere of the average fact finder's experience or knowledge. It is the expert's specialized knowledge, skill, experience, and training that unlock the gateway to the courtroom. Notably, the relevance and reliability of an expert's opinion are the *sine qua non* of admission into trial proceedings. Whether a particular jurisdiction adheres to *Daubert* or *Frye* admissibility standards, it behooves the proffered expert to provide opinions that conform to the applicable standard in order to survive the scrutiny of the judicial gatekeeper. To the extent possible, expert opinions should be expressed to the degree of certainty required by the jurisdiction where the opinion is to be offered.

REFERENCES

1. Phillmore JG. *The History and Principles of the Law of Evidence: As Illustrating Our Social Progress*. London: Benning & Co; 1850.
2. Pacia RA, Pacia RA. Roman contributions to American civil jurisprudence. *Rhode Island Bar Journal*. 2001; 49: 5.
3. Langbein JH. Historical foundations of the law of evidence: a view from the Ryder Sources. *Columbia Law Review*. 1996; 96: 1168–1202.
4. Golan T. Revisiting the history of scientific expert testimony. *Brooklyn Law Review*. 2008; 73(3): 879–942.
5. Hand L. Historical and practical considerations regarding expert testimony. *Harvard Law Review*. 1901; 15(1): 40–58.
6. *Frye v. U.S.*, 293 F. 1013 (D.C. Cir 1923).
7. Mnookin JL. Idealizing science and demonizing experts: an intellectual history of expert evidence. *Villanova Law Review*. 2007; 52(4): 763–802.
8. Oldham JC. The origins of the special jury. *University of Chicago Law Review*. 1983; 50(1): 137–221.
9. *Folkes v. Chadd*, 99 Eng. Rep. 589 (1782).
10. Landsman S. One hundred years of rectitude: medical witnesses at the Old Bailey, 1717–1817. *Law and History Review*. 1998; 16(3): 445–494.
11. Friedman LM. Expert testimony, its abuse and reformation. *Yale Law Journal*. 1910; 19(4): 247–257.
12. Clearwater AT. Medical expert testimony. *The North American Review*. 1909; 189(643): 821–830.
13. New York State Bar Association. *Proceedings of the Thirty-Second Annual Meeting of the New York State Bar*. Albany: The Argus Company; 1909.
14. Golan T. *Laws of Men and Laws of Nature: The History of Scientific Expert Testimony in England and America*. Cambridge, MA: Harvard University Press; 2004.
15. Horton TM. The debate is over: *Frye* lives no more. *Thurgood Marshall Law Review*. 1994; 19(2): 379–400.
16. Dillhoff M. Science, law, and truth: defining the scope of the *Daubert* trilogy. *Notre Dame Law Review*. 2011; 86(3): 1289–1318.
17. Morgan EM. Practical difficulties impeding reform in the law of evidence. *Vanderbilt Law Review*. 1961; 14(3): 725–740.
18. Ladd M. A modern code of evidence. *Iowa Law Review*. 1942; 27(2): 213–231.
19. Fed. R. Evid. 702 (1975).

20. Chan EJ. The "Brave New World" of *Daubert*: true peer review, editorial peer review, and scientific validity. *NYU Law Review*. 1995; 70(1): 100–134.
21. Giannelli PC. The admissibility of novel scientific evidence: *Frye v. United States*, a half-century later. *Columbia Law Review*. 1980; 80: 1197–1250.
22. Fed. R. Evid. 402 (1975).
23. Huber P. Medical experts and the ghost of Galileo. *Law and Contemporary Problems*. 1991; 54(3): 119–170.
24. Elliot ED. Toward incentive-based procedure: three approaches for regulating scientific evidence. *Boston University Law Review*. 1989; 69(3): 487–512, at 492.
25. *Daubert v. Merrell Dow Pharmaceuticals*, 509 U.S. 579 (1993).
26. *General Electric Co. v. Joiner*, 522 U.S. 136 (1997).
27. *Kumho Tire Co., Ltd. v. Carmichael*, 526 U.S. 137 (1999).
28. Goodwin RJ. Fifty years of *Frye* in Alabama: the continuing debate over adopting the test established in *Daubert v. Merrell Dow Pharmaceuticals, Inc. Cumberland Law Review*. 2004; 35(2): 231–316.
29. *U.S. v. Addison*, 498 F.2d 741, 744 (1974).
30. Simmons R. Conquering the province of the jury: expert testimony and the professionalization of fact-finding. *University of Cincinnati Law Review*. 2006; 74(3): 1013–1066.
31. *U.S. v. Rincon*, 28 F.3d 921 (9th Cir. 1994).
32. Rappeport JR. Reasonable medical certainty. *Bull Am Acad Psychiatry Law*. 1985; 13(1): 5–15.
33. Lewin JL. The genesis and evolution of legal uncertainty about "Reasonable Medical Certainty." *Maryland Law Review*. 1998; 57: 380–504.
34. Hullverson JE. Reasonable degree of medical certainty: A Tort et a Travers. *St. Louis University Law Journal*. 1987; 31(3): 577–598.
35. Diamond BL. Reasonable medical certainty, diagnostic thresholds, and definitions of mental illness in the legal context. *Bull Am Acad Psychiatry Law*. 1985: 13(2): 121–128.

CHAPTER 2

Criminal Culpability: A Developmental Approach

NICOLE FOUBISTER AND FRANK K. TEDESCHI

Throughout history, human civilization has sought to define the age at which a person achieves maturity and responsibility. Regardless of the epoch or culture, certain characteristics have been employed in determining at what point a juvenile becomes an adult, including the ability to reason, to understand the consequences of one's behaviors, and to exert control over one's actions. Although courts, politicians, theologians, and scholars may have differed as to the precise age of majority, society has tried to distinguish childhood from adulthood. Inherent in this concept is the notion of legal culpability, such that a person becoming an adult is legally accountable for his or her behavior.

Developmental neuroscience and psychology have played increasingly prominent roles in court proceedings involving juvenile offenders. Research has demonstrated that adolescents may be more impulsive, less able to exert emotional control, and more sensation seeking than adults. This has led many to argue that adolescents are less culpable than adults who commit the same crime, much in the way that individuals with mental illness and intellectual disabilities are seen as less blameworthy. The U.S. Supreme Court has affirmed this view in several important cases, which cited specific developmental research findings in issuing their rulings.

Child and adolescent forensic psychiatry has become intimately involved in the process of juvenile justice, not only in the treatment and rehabilitation of juvenile delinquents but also in informing the court about the latest research on adolescent development and subsequent questions of culpability.

In this chapter, we will review current research in adolescent development and its application in expert testimony regarding juvenile culpability. We will begin with a review of current research in neurobiologic, cognitive, and psychosocial models of adolescent development and the characteristics of juvenile delinquents. Next, we will discuss the use of these models in examining adolescent culpability and case precedents. Finally, we will outline the evaluation of adolescent culpability and areas of focus in expert testimony, as well as areas of likely challenge under cross-examination.

ADOLESCENT DEVELOPMENT AND CULPABILITY: WHAT DO WE KNOW?

Neurobiologic and Neuroanatomic Models of Adolescence Development

At the most basic level, in early adolescence dopamine transmission and activity increases in multiple regions of the brain.[1,2] Dopamine mediates reward and behavioral reinforcement, and the areas in which dopaminergic transmission increases around puberty are associated with a number of social information processing functions, as well as reward processing.[1,2] As a result the dopaminergic system becomes much more sensitive and efficient, heightening not only the experience of a reward but also giving it greater salience in a context where both reward and risk are present.[2,3] This in turn leads to greater risk taking in adolescents, as well as "sensation seeking" in which rewards are preferentially sought due to the greater experience of pleasure provided via these sensitized dopaminergic pathways.[2,4] Social interaction with peers becomes rewarding in a way that was not previously present in childhood, with evidence that in adolescence social acceptance is processed similarly to other types of rewards.[2,5,6]

Structurally, two key processes occur during adolescence that affect numerous neural circuits. The first is a reduction in gray matter density in the frontal and parietal regions of the brain due to a pruning of unused synaptic connections.[7,8] This process allows for more efficient information processing and the creation of greater specialization of brain regions, such as areas of the prefrontal cortex.[9,10] This change in gray matter density is directly related to the improvements in cognitive abilities, reasoning, and memory seen in early adolescence.[11,12] Areas of the frontal lobes and prefrontal cortex are among the last to show evidence of this synaptic pruning in late adolescence and early adulthood.[1,9,13] It is these areas of the brain that permit behavioral inhibition in emotional responses to a stimulus, weighing the rewards and risks of a situation, and planning and executing a response.[14,15] In the second process there is a gradual myelination of the neural tracts between areas of cortical gray matter, allowing for more rapid and efficient transmission of neural impulses and facilitating the development of more fully integrated brain activity.[15] Although an over-all increase in white matter density and volume occurs as the brain matures,[11] there are differences in the timing and rates of myelination in different brain regions.[16] Unlike gray matter pruning, which starts in early adolescence and is largely complete by midadolescence, myelination of the prefrontal cortex begins in childhood and continues into early adulthood or even later.[17-19] This proliferation of white matter in the prefrontal cortex enhances and strengthens the effects of the prior refinement of connectivity that was achieved through synaptic pruning and translates to further progress in the ability to make complicated decisions, plan ahead, and weigh risks and rewards.[4]

These changes in brain structure and efficiency directly influence the functioning of what Steinberg has called "a tale of two brain systems," which are employed to differing degrees during different stages of adolescence in motivating and regulating behaviors.[2] The predominant system in early and midadolescence is referred to as the *socioemotional system*, which processes social and emotional information, as well as the experience of reward and punishment. The socioemotional system is composed of the brain regions that undergo dopaminergic remodeling at the onset of puberty and mediate risk-taking and sensation-seeking behaviors. In contrast, the *cognitive control system* is the system that governs executive functioning, impulse control, the evaluation of risks and rewards, planning, and a perception of the future. It is created through the myelination of connections both within and between brain structures and is completed in the mid-20s.[2]

While young children and early adolescents have the ability to employ impulse control, it is only with the maturation of the cognitive control system that impulse control can be more consistently used.[15] The key fact in understanding the differing weights that the socioemotional and cognitive control systems have at different ages is the disjunction in the onset of their actions, with the socioemotional system dominating in early and midadolescence and the cognitive control system fully exerting its effects in late adolescence and early adulthood.[1,2,14] For this reason, in early and midadolescence the socio-emotional system drives more reckless and impulsive behaviors in the context of an immature and less effective cognitive control system. This period of time has been likened to "starting the engines with an unskilled driver" (p. 17).[20] Given the high sensitivity to and salience of reward, more emotionally motivated behaviors, and greater susceptibility to peer influence, it is during this developmental stage that adolescents are particularly vulnerable to engaging in delinquent behaviors. As myelination proceeds through late adolescence and the 20s, self-regulation becomes more efficient and effective, judgment and impulse control improve, and the dopaminergic reward systems become less sensitized.[14]

Cognitive Models of Adolescence Development

The aforementioned changes to gray matter, white matter, and connectivity act to shape the adolescent brain to one that is progressively more capable of complex cognitive tasks, which affects decision making. As a result, by age 16, most individuals have achieved an adult level of competence on cognitive tasks that primarily employ the frontal lobes, in particular the prefrontal cortex.[2] This includes the domains of working memory, the estimation of future outcomes, verbal fluency, response inhibition, deductive reasoning, and processing speed.[2,21-25] Due to more efficient processing, greater comprehension, and markedly improved ability to reason, by midadolescence teenagers have the capability to engage in multidimensional and abstract thinking, as well as to consider hypothetical scenarios and responses.[26]

However, one must keep in mind that these measures of cognitive abilities in adolescence are experimental in nature and do not recreate real-world decision making shaped by emotional context and family, peer, and societal influence, and where the potential rewards of a decision have a disproportionate salience over negative consequences. It has been posited that adolescents' judgment not only is derived from their cognitive capacities but is also significantly more influenced by emotional and social variables than that of adults.[1] As a result of the conflict that may frequently arise between cognition and psychosocial factors, adolescents may be less able to effectively use their cognitive capabilities to exercise good judgment.

Related to the adolescent decision-making process are the concepts of "hot cognition" and "cool cognition."[16,20] "Hot cognition" refers to thought processes that occur under conditions of high arousal or strong emotion; "cool cognition" describes those that occur in situations of low arousal and low emotional content. Under experimental "cool cognition" conditions, adolescents are able to perform at adult competency levels in tests of cognition and decision making. However, some researchers believe that due to the neurobiologic changes previously discussed, adolescents are particularly susceptible to emotional factors in their decisions in real life, which leads to more frequent use of "hot cognition" and the adverse consequences that can result. It has also been suggested that in determining risk, adolescents tend to focus on and overestimate the quantitative aspects of rewards and put less emphasis on potential negative outcomes of behaviors as adults do.[27] Also, adolescents tend to be less future-oriented when making decisions and may disregard consequences due to a lack of life experience.[28-30]

Psychosocial Models of Adolescent Development

Social interaction and peer affiliation during adolescence take on an importance that is unmatched in childhood and adulthood, which in part is related to an increase in the number of oxytocin receptors in limbic structures.[2,31] In considering the role of peer influences on behaviors and decision making, it is important to note that psychosocial maturity develops much more slowly than cognitive maturity. It has been demonstrated that when in groups, risk taking significantly increases in adolescents, and resistance to peer influence is lowest in early adolescence.[32,33] Antisocial peer influence therefore has its greatest effect in early adolescence, with evidence that juveniles are far more likely to commit crimes together in groups than adults.[34] Between ages 14 and 18, resistance to peer influence linearly increases, secondary to a declining sensitivity to social rewards and reward salience, as well as the development of an integrated sense of self.[1,2] Peer pressure may influence adolescent decision making through direct coercion by peers or indirectly through adolescents' fear that they will be rejected if they do not comply with the demands of their group. There is some additional evidence that antisocial conduct and more risky behaviors may confer a higher status among peers.[35]

In addition, adolescents appear inherently less able to maintain self-regulation. Impulsivity is distinct from sensation seeking in that the former stems from diminished self-control (via an immature cognitive control system), while the latter is secondary to a willingness to seek out novel stimuli that may be rewarding (via an active socioemotional system).[16] The ability to exert self-control and diminish impulsivity has been demonstrated to increase linearly from early adolescence well into adulthood.[36,37]

21ST-CENTURY CASE PRECEDENT INVOLVING THE DIMINISHED RESPONSIBILITY OF ADOLESCENTS

In the landmark case *Roper v. Simmons* (2005) it was argued that because the U.S. Supreme Court had ruled that the death penalty for persons with mental retardation was cruel and unusual, the principle should also be applied to juveniles, as they were also less culpable than adults and less able to deliberate their actions.[38,39] The Court agreed with this contention and affirmed that the death penalty for juveniles younger than 18 was a violation of the Eighth and Fourteenth Amendments.[40] The Court's decision was derived from a recognition of a national and international consensus against the imposition of a juvenile death penalty and was also heavily influenced by research in adolescent development, which attested to the distinctiveness of adolescent offenders and their lesser culpability due to their developmental immaturity.

The ruling in *Roper* also opened the door to the use of neuroscientific and developmental research in considering the constitutionality of other severe adult sentences for juvenile offenders. Five years later, in *Graham v. Florida* (2010) and its companion case *Sullivan v. Florida* (2010), the Court examined the imposition of life sentences without parole for nonhomicide crimes committed by juveniles.[41,42] Neuroscience was even more explicitly relied upon by the Court in *Graham*, which used the same logic and neuroscientific arguments as in *Roper*: that life sentences without parole for juvenile nonhomicide offenses were categorically cruel and unusual due to the lesser culpability of adolescents and are prohibited by the Eighth and Fourteenth Amendments.[41]

In *Miller v. Alabama* (2012) and *Jackson v. Hobbs* (2012) the Court further extended the rationales of adolescent diminished responsibility, "lessened culpability," and "capacity for change" that had been employed in *Roper* and *Graham* in holding that mandatory life without parole for juveniles who had committed homicide was also a constitutional violation.[43,44] The *Miller* ruling, however, did not require retroactivity. Thus, some states have adopted procedures for resentencing of offenders in mandatory-life situations, whereas others are regarding only new cases. The resentencing hearings have been a fertile area for expert testimony about adolescent brain development.

EXPERT TESTIMONY AND AREAS OF CHALLENGE TO TESTIMONY

The Expert Evaluation of Adolescent Culpability

The role of the expert witness' assessment and testimony in cases where the degree of a juvenile's culpability is in question can be pertinent in several judicial settings and phases of a trial.[45] These include:

- Negotiation between the defense and prosecution regarding the appropriate charge
- Waiver of adolescents to adult criminal court
- The guilt phase of a trial
- Disposition of adolescents who have been found delinquent in juvenile court
- The penalty phase in adult criminal court

Both in the forensic report to the court and in testimony to the fact finder, the expert must specifically and unambiguously lay out how developmental factors may have contributed to mitigation or affect proportionality. As with all expert testimony, the *Frye* and *Daubert* standards must be carefully observed; they are particularly important with regard to adolescent research and neuroimaging studies, as what is accepted within the field and supported by the literature is continually evolving and is at times controversial.

As we have discussed, there is abundant evidence from psychological, neurobiologic, and developmental research, as well as legal precedent, that an adolescent may be considered less culpable than an adult who commits the same offense. The difficulty lies, however, in evaluating whether a *particular* child or adolescent is less blameworthy for a *particular* criminal act than an adult charged with the same crime. This is the question posed to the expert by judges and attorneys. Forensic assessments of juvenile culpability are multifaceted. The evaluation must incorporate opinions on psychiatric diagnoses and the potential for rehabilitation of the defendant and must determine how an individual adolescent's behavior matches up with age-specific developmental models. As outlined by Peter Ash, the evaluation of adolescent culpability is recommended to include 10 separate factors in reaching an opinion.[45] These factors may have areas of overlap and can synergistically interact both to reduce or enhance culpability. They are:

1. *Appreciation of wrongfulness*—Was there an intellectual or social deficit that prevented the juvenile from understanding that his or her behaviors were wrong? Acute mental illnesses (most notably psychosis) at the time of the offense must be given attention in this area.

2. *Ability to conform to the law*—Could the juvenile refrain from committing the offense? Were there neurobiologic, psychological, cognitive, and/or social factors that led to excessive impulsivity, failure to make the right decisions, or enhanced suggestibility?

3. *Developmental course of aggression*—Were aggressive acts primarily in the context of interactions with peers or instead perpetrated alone? Is there a history of serious violent offenses? Did aggression begin at a younger age? A more longstanding and pervasive pattern of aggression that began at an early age is likely to be more difficult to rehabilitate.

4. *Immaturity*—Areas in evaluating immaturity that may be included are psychometric assessments of IQ and cognitive functioning, susceptibility to peer pressure, psychosocial maturity, ability to empathize, tendency to engage in risk taking, and a sense of time and the future. If a juvenile's capacity to make decisions is not substantially different from an adult's or that of a same-age peer, diminished responsibility should not apply.

5. *Out-of-character action*—Did the offender act out of character with regard to the expectations that society places on juveniles? This relates to the principle of what a "reasonable adolescent" would do in a given situation that led to the criminal act—was it a gross departure from typical adolescent behavior (robbery, rape, arson)?

6. *Environmental circumstances*—Poverty, high-crime neighborhoods, and living with family members who are abusive or encourage antisocial attitudes are each associated with higher rates of juvenile delinquency. Many of the environmental influences in a juvenile's life are out of his or her control to avoid. This is a key area of difference with adults that the Supreme Court recognized in *Roper*.[38] Data on the effects of abuse, poverty, family structure, and community influence on adolescent behavior may be incorporated in supporting the expert's ultimate opinion.

7. *Peer group norms*—There are data suggesting that appearing weak in a group of peers or attempting to resist their influence can have severe consequences, such as being socially ostracized or targeted for victimization.[46] Aggression and violence that are justified and may be adaptive in such groups can be seen by youths as less reprehensible, despite the fact that they may have a sense that the broader culture views such behaviors as criminal.[45] Care must be used not to extend these considerations to individuals who choose to affiliate with deviant peer groups such as gangs, where criminal behavior is the norm.

8. *Incomplete personality development*—Developmental theory posits that adolescence is a time of identity consolidation and a juvenile's personality may significantly change with time. As adolescents' personality is not yet fixed, it can be argued that their criminal behaviors have not resulted from an inherently "bad" character, and as a result they should be held less responsible for an act that does not stem from a fully developed criminal identity. This is an area that can be particularly problematic for the expert, as the field cannot yet reliably distinguish between what Moffitt has referred to as "adolescent-limited" and "life-course-persistent" offenders,[35] a limitation that the Supreme Court specifically referenced in its rulings in *Roper* and *Graham*.[38,41]

9. *Mental illness*—The expert should thoroughly assess the juvenile for psychiatric illness using standard assessment tools and updated *DSM-5* diagnostic criteria, and clearly delineate in his or her evaluation and testimony any connection between the adolescent's mental illness and the perpetration of the crime if present.

10. *Reactive attitudes toward the offense*—This refers to the reactions that one has to another's behavior in response to an assessment of his or her intent.[45] If an adolescent's offense is viewed with adult intentionality, he or she will be held to a higher degree of culpability; if the behavior is felt to result from a child's intent, he or she can be seen as less culpable.

Challenges to Testimony

1. The limits of neuroscience

As research in child and adolescent neurobiology has advanced, prosecutors and attorneys are increasingly introducing neuroscience as evidence for or against juvenile culpability in criminal trials.[47] Behavioral research tends to be given more credibility when accompanied by a neurobiologic explanation and in a recent study was shown to have an influence on judges' decisions in criminal cases.[14,48] But while research in neuroscience is a seductive means of attempting to explain a juvenile's behavior, there are clear limits to what it can tell us. First, one must keep in mind that the research actually provides *aggregate* data that represent *trends* in developmental trajectories among a large number of individuals. This allows the expert to make generalizations about brain maturation and functional capability in youths based on averages of data but says little about a particular individual's brain. There is simply too much variation between even same-age individuals, let alone across ages or developmental stages, to assert that any one adolescent's brain is any more or less mature than another's.[14,47,49] Second, even among averaged data there is no clear point at which the adolescent brain can be said to have made the transition to an adult brain.[14] Third, there are no current universally accepted and reliable methods by which all dimensions of neurobiologic immaturity can be measured on an individual basis.[45,47] In light of these limitations, the most appropriate use of neuroscience by the expert is to inform the fact finders of general maturational processes known to occur in childhood and adolescence and the behavioral, cognitive, and psychological outcomes that *could* result from those processes.

2. The limits of neuroimaging

Neuroimaging is a particularly alluring option for evidence of diminished responsibility, as it is viewed as "hard" scientific evidence even among other neurobiologic and behavioral research.[15] An image from a particular individual's brain may be proffered in court to illustrate that activation or decreased activity of a particular anatomic region is associated with a specific behavior. Although research studies have gone to great lengths to point out that the association between patterns of brain activation and cognitive or behavioral processes are correlational, these findings are often misinterpreted as causal.[13] In addition, this type of research is still at a stage of relative infancy.

3. The reliability of measures of the psychosocial maturity of the juvenile offender

If one accepts that juvenile culpability exists on a continuum and can be affected by aspects of psychosocial maturity, such as the tendency to take risks, ability to exert impulse control, and degree of resistance to peer influence, then it becomes important to in some way assess these attributes in a given juvenile offender. Within the fields of psychology and psychiatry there are no standardized scales that can be employed to quantify a child or adolescent's psychosocial maturity or the degree to which his or her identity has consolidated on an individual basis.[45,50] We have the ability to measure the cognitive and intellectual capacities of individuals through psychological testing, but these results do not address issues of maturity. However, information in the domains of psychosocial maturity can still be obtained, and this is important to investigate. This can be accomplished through the forensic clinical interview, which can explore aspects of psychosocial maturity such as the ability to exert emotional control, the degree of influence of the environment, resilience and independence, the ability to take others' perspectives, and the individual's appreciation of the consequences of his or her actions. In addition, collecting collateral information in these areas from individuals who know the subject well may be useful, such as family, school staff, and medical professionals.

4. Distinguishing adolescent-limited from repeat juvenile offenders

The vast majority of juvenile offenders do not continue to engage in antisocial behaviors as adults.[1,35,50-52] However, 5% to 10% of juvenile offenders fall into Moffitt's "life-course-persistent offender" group, who go on to engage in criminal behaviors throughout their life.[1,35,51] Criminal behaviors that manifest in the "adolescent-limited" group arise as the product of the process of identity formation and experimentation in different behaviors and are much more amenable to rehabilitation.[35,42] Those of the life-course-persistent offender group, in contrast, reflect an identity that is not "unformed" but has instead already consolidated into a behavioral pattern of criminality, which may be more resistant to attempts to rehabilitate it.[35,51] It is currently beyond the ability of any evaluator to reliably differentiate between these two types of offenders. This is likely to be an area of challenge to testimony, as the models of lesser culpability and mitigation for juvenile offenders are based on science and research that pertain to the adolescent-limited population rather than the life-course-persistent population.

5. Why don't all juveniles engage in criminal behaviors?

A self-report study found that 80% to 90% of adolescent boys surveyed admitted to committing a crime for which they could be incarcerated.[50] The majority of crimes committed tend to be relatively minor, and the typical juvenile does not continue to engage in illegal behaviors into adulthood. The likelihood of repeat offenses is determined by the relative balance of delinquency risk and protective factors, which will vary for every individual and are a vital part of a juvenile forensic psychiatric evaluation.

6. Previous emphasis of data that pertain to normal development

To date, the U.S. Supreme Court has relied on research that has described *normal* development in considering issues of child and adolescent criminal culpability; however, there are multiple distinctions between the general population and juvenile delinquents, including differences in rates of mental illness, history of trauma, and intellectual and cognitive abilities, which are associated with *pathological* development. The data from research investigating normal development may not adequately generalize to juvenile delinquents. In the near future, research on pathological development in the context of cognitive deficits and psychiatric diagnoses may be used in arguments of lesser culpability and mitigation.

7. Why immaturity can't be used in adult culpability defenses

The argument cannot be made that adults who are impulsive and lack an appreciation of the consequences of their actions are less blameworthy or less culpable for their actions in the same way as an adolescent. In the case of adult criminals, although their behaviors may appear similar, they are instead often "characterological" and are enduring traits of a formed personality that are unlikely to change with the passage of time.[1,50] In this way for adults there is a connection between a "bad act" and "bad character" that is not present for most adolescents.

8. The balance between adolescent responsibility and lesser culpability

The argument that juveniles can be less culpable as a result of normal developmental processes should not be misinterpreted as a statement that adolescents are not responsible for their actions. While it can be argued that mitigation and proportionality should be applied in certain cases, adolescents must still be held responsible for their criminal behaviors. In the case of older, violent recidivists, many should be tried and sentenced as adults, as their culpability is nearly at an adult level and their behaviors are less likely to be normative compared to the adolescent who is caught smoking marijuana or shoplifting.[35,50] The purpose of the models of diminished juvenile responsibility is not to remove punishment, but to modulate it in a manner that appropriately takes into account the developmental processes that set adolescents apart from adults. It is this balance between serving the societal need for justice and applying it appropriately to youth that juvenile justice policy attempts to achieve.

THE IMPORTANCE OF REHABILITATION

To complete this discussion, one must consider the effects that being tried and incarcerated as an adult may have on the developmental trajectory and mental health of an adolescent. If, as Moffitt has posited, criminal behaviors are confined to adolescence in nearly 9 out of 10 juveniles,[35,51] does incarceration serve the goals of deterrence and rehabilitation, or does it instead push adolescents toward a life-persistent pattern of criminality?

Unfortunately, the accumulated evidence suggests that the latter scenario is true. If the incarceration of adolescents in adult correctional facilities has contributed to the decrease in juvenile felony rates seen since the mid-1990s, it appears it has done so through incapacitation alone, rather than through deterrence or rehabilitation.[50] Multiple studies have illustrated that juveniles sentenced in the adult criminal court have recidivism rates that are substantially increased, with a greater likelihood of rearrest for felonies that ranges from 26.5% to 77%.[53] Juveniles who are incarcerated in adult facilities are also more likely to reoffend more quickly and more frequently.[54] It has also been demonstrated that longer sentences do not have an effect on deterrence or reducing recidivism.[54,55]

Juvenile offenders who already have higher baseline rates of trauma are more likely to be victimized both physically and sexually in jails and prisons.[54] Both the modeling of antisocial behaviors and the threat of repeated trauma during incarceration are likely to severely disrupt normal social and emotional development. Juveniles are also more likely to receive inadequate psychiatric treatment, as psychiatric services in adult institutions are not designed to treat adolescents.[56] As a result of incarceration, access to education and vocational skills training is limited, which reduces the likelihood that the juvenile will find gainful employment once his or her sentence is finished.[1] Taken together, the data suggest that incarceration for juveniles in adult settings exacerbates criminal behavior through aberrant social development, traumatization, and inadequately treated psychiatric illness and by limiting the options for prosocial behaviors following release due to inadequate education and difficulty entering the labor force.

Despite this grim assessment of the effects of incarceration in adult settings, research has shown that meaningful rehabilitation of juvenile offenders can be achieved in both institutional and community settings. The programs that have been found to be most effective in reducing recidivism are those that employ knowledge of adolescent development, provide a supportive environment, and focus on improving social skills, self-control, academic performance, and vocational skills.[1,57] Such programs include the acquisition of anger management and conflict resolution skills (Interpersonal Skills Training), the use of an authoritative adult who acts as a "teaching parent" (Teaching Family Homes), and modified cognitive-behavior therapy (CBT) programs.[58] These interventions have been associated with significant decreases in recidivism, ranging from 30% to 35%.[58] Multisystemic therapy, which addresses risk factors in multiple domains, incorporates CBT, parent training, and family therapy and in some studies has been found to reduce recidivism by 50% in the community setting.[59] Each of these interventions not only has a large effect size but is also substantially less expensive than incarceration.[50]

The current literature suggests that for the majority of juvenile offenders, the application of criminal sentences in adult correctional facilities is not indicated, particularly for nonviolent juvenile offenders. There appears to be limited benefit of such punitive measures in rehabilitating the individual or ultimately to society. The need for punishment remains, but punishment should be balanced with an effort to protect a juvenile's transition to adulthood, as this too serves the needs of society. It may be that this balance will best be achieved within the juvenile justice system rather than in the adult corrections system, as originally envisioned by the reform movements of the 19th century. Juvenile correctional facilities are able to meet the need for punishment and incapacitation but are also better poised to enact developmentally informed rehabilitative programs in an infrastructure specifically designed for adolescents. To effect such change legislative reform and the revision of statutory sentencing guidelines must occur. If we are to adhere to the mission of protecting those who are less blameworthy and less culpable, this task is as important as providing testimony in court, and will require continued advocacy and guidance from mental health professionals who are dedicated to this vulnerable population.

REFERENCES

1. Steinberg L. Adolescent development and juvenile justice. *Ann Rev Clin Psychol.* 2009; 5: 459–485.

2. Steinberg L. A social neuroscience perspective on adolescent risk-taking. *Dev Rev.* 2008; 28(1): 78–106.

3. Ernst M, Speak L. Reward systems. In: de Haan M, Gunnar M, eds. *Handbook of Developmental Social Neuroscience.* New York: Guilford Press; 2009: 324–341.

4. Steinberg L. Does recent research on adolescent brain development inform the mature minor doctrine? *J Med Philos.* 2013; 38(3): 256–267.

5. Galvan A, Hare TA, Davidson M, Spicer J, Glover G, Casey BJ. The role of ventral frontostriatal circuitry in reward-based learning in humans. *J Neurosci.* 2005; 25(38): 8650–8656.

6. May JC, Delgado MR, Dahl RE, et al. Event-related functional magnetic resonance imaging of reward-related brain circuitry in children and adolescents. *Biol Psychiat.* 2004; 55(4): 359–366.

7. Sowell ER, Thompson PM, Tessner KD, Toga AW. Mapping continued brain growth and gray matter density reduction in dorsal frontal cortex: Inverse relationships during postadolescent brain maturation. *J Neurosci.* 2001; 21(22): 8819–8829.

8. Gogtay N, Giedd JN, Lusk L, et al. Dynamic mapping of human cortical development during childhood through early adulthood. *Proc Natl Acad Sci USA.* 2004; 101(21): 8174–8179.

9. Gogtay N, Thompson PM. Mapping gray matter development: implications for typical development and vulnerability to psychopathology. *Brain Cognition.* 2010; 72(1): 6–15.

10. Casey BJ, Trainor RJ, Orendi JL, et al. A developmental functional MRI study of prefrontal activation during performance of a go-no-go task. *J Cogn Neurosci.* 1997; 9(6): 835–847.

11. Giedd JN. The teen brain: insights from neuroimaging. *J Adolesc Health.* 2008; 42(4): 335–343.

12. Luciana M, Conklin HM, Hooper CJ, Yarger RS. The development of nonverbal working memory and executive control processes in adolescents. *Child Dev.* 2005; 76(3): 697–712.

13. Aronson JD. Brain imaging, culpability and the juvenile death penalty. *Psychol Public Pol Law.* 2007; 13(2): 115–142.

14. Steinberg L. Should the science of adolescent brain development inform public policy? *Am Psychol.* 2009; 64(8): 739–750.

15. Johnson SB, Blum RW, Giedd JN. Adolescent maturity and the brain: the promise and pitfalls of neuroscience research in adolescent health policy. *J Adolesc Health.* 2009; 45(3): 216–221.

16. Kambam P, Thompson C. The development of decision-making capacities in children and adolescents: psychological and neurological perspectives and their implications for juvenile defendants. *Behav Sci Law.* 2009; 27(2): 173–190.

17. Bartzokis G, Beckson M, Lu PH, Nuechterlein KH, Edwards N, Mintz J. Age-related changes in frontal and temporal lobe volumes in men: a magnetic resonance imaging study. *Arch Gen Psychiat.* 2001; 58: 461–465.

18. Lenroot RK, Gogtay N, Greensteinet DK, et al. Sexual dimorphism of brain developmental trajectories during childhood and adolescence. *Neuroimage.* 2007; 36(4): 1065–1073.

19. Barnea-Goraly N, Menon V, Eckert M, et al. White matter development during childhood and adolescence: a cross-sectional diffusion tensor imaging study. *Cereb Cortex.* 2005; 15(12): 1848–1854.

20. Dahl RE. Adolescent brain development: A period of vulnerabilities and opportunities. Keynote address. *Ann NY Acad Sci.* 2004; 1021(1): 1–22.
21. Conklin HM, Luciana M, Hooper CJ, Yarger RS. Working memory performance in typically developing children and adolescents: behavioral evidence of protracted frontal lobe development. *Dev Neuropsychol.* 2007; 31(1): 103–128.
22. Crone EA, van der Molen MW. Developmental changes in real-life decision making: performance on a gambling task previously shown to depend on the ventromedial prefrontal cortex. *Dev Neuropsychol.* 2004; 25(3): 251–279.
23. Luna B, Thulborn KR, Munoz DP, et al. Maturation of widely distributed brain function subserves cognitive development. *Neuroimage.* 2001; 13(5): 786–793.
24. Hooper CJ, Luciana M, Conklin HM, Yarger RS. Adolescents' performance on the Iowa Gambling Task: implications for the development of decision making and ventromedial prefrontal cortex. *Dev Psychol.* 2004; 40(6): 1148–1158.
25. Hale S. A global developmental trend in cognitive processing speed. *Child Dev.* 1990; 61(3): 653–663.
26. Kuhn D. Adolescent thinking. In: Lerner R, Steinberg L, eds. *Handbook of Adolescent Psychology.* 3rd ed. New York: Wiley; 2009: 152–186.
27. Reyna VF, Estrada SM, DeMarinis JA, Myers RM, Stanisz JM, Mills BA. Neurobiological and memory models of risky decision making in adolescents versus young adults. *J Exp Psychol Learn.* 2011; 37(5): 1125–1142.
28. Steinberg L, Albert D, Cauffman E, Banich M, Graham S, Woolard J. Age differences in sensation seeking and impulsivity as indexed by behavior and self-report: evidence for a dual systems model. *Dev Psychol.* 2008; 44(6): 1764–1778.
29. Feld BC. Competence, culpability, and punishment: implications of *Atkins* for executing and sentencing adolescents. *Hofstra Law Review.* 2003; 32: 463–552.
30. Reppucci ND. Adolescent development and juvenile justice. *Am J Commun Psychol.* 1999; 27(3): 307–326.
31. Spear LP. The adolescent brain and age-related behavioral manifestations. *Neurosci Biobehav Rev.* 2000; 24(4): 417–463.
32. Gardner M, Steinberg L. Peer influence on risk taking, risk preference, and risky decision making in adolescence and adulthood: An experimental study. *Dev Psychol.* 2005; 41(4): 625–635.
33. Steinberg L, Monahan KC. Age differences in resistance to peer influence. *Dev Psychol.* 2007; 43(6): 1531–1543.
34. Zimring FE. *American Youth Violence.* New York: Oxford University Press; 2000.
35. Moffitt TE. Adolescence-limited and life-course-persistent antisocial behavior: a developmental taxonomy. *Psychol Rev.* 1993; 100(4): 674–701.
36. Zuckerman M. *Sensation Seeking: Beyond the Optimal Level of Arousal.* Hillsdale, NJ: Erlbaum; 1979.
37. Galvan A, Hare T, Voss H, Glover G, Casey BJ. Risk-taking and the adolescent brain: who is at risk?. *Dev Sci.* 2007; 10(2): F8–F14.
38. *Roper v. Simmons*, 543 U.S. 551, 125 S. Ct. 1183, 161 L. Ed. 2d 1 (2005).
39. Siegel DM. The Supreme Court and the sentencing of juveniles in the United States: reaffirming the distinctiveness of youth. *Child Adolesc Psych Clin.* 2011; 20(3): 431–445.
40. Scott CL. *Roper v. Simmons*: can juvenile offenders be executed?. *J Am Acad Psychiatry.* 2005; 33(4): 547–552.
41. *Graham v. Florida*, 130 S. Ct. 2011, 560 U.S. 48, 176 L. Ed. 2d 825 (2010).
42. *Sullivan v. Florida*, 130 S. Ct. 2059 (2010).

43. *Miller v. Alabama*, 132 S. Ct. 2455, 567 U.S., 183 L. Ed. 2d 407 (2012).

44. *Jackson v. Hobbs*, 132 S. Ct. 548, 181 L. Ed. 2d 395 (2011).

45. Ash P. But he knew it was wrong: evaluating adolescent culpability. *J Am Acad Psychiatry.* 2012; 40(1): 21–32.

46. Fagan J. Contexts of choice by adolescents in criminal events. In: Grisso T, Schwartz R, eds. *Youth on Trial.* Chicago, IL: University of Chicago Press; 2000: 371–402.

47. Bonnie RJ, Scott ES. The teenage brain: adolescent brain research and the law. *Curr Dir Psychol Sci.* 2013; 22(2): 158–161.

48. Aspinwall LG, Brown TR, Tabery J. The double-edged sword: Does biomechanism increase or decrease judges' sentencing of psychopaths? *Science.* 2012; 337(6096): 846–849.

49. Maroney TA. Adolescent brain science after *Graham v. Florida. Notre Dame Law Review.* 2011; 86: 765–794.

50. Scott ES, Steinberg L. Adolescent development and the regulation of youth crime. *Future Child.* 2008; 18(2): 15–33.

51. Moffitt TE, Caspi A, Harrington H, Milne BJ. Males on the life-course-persistent and adolescence-limited antisocial pathways: follow-up at age 26 years. *Dev Psychopathol.* 2002; 14(1): 179–207.

52. Piquero AR, Farrington DP, Blumstein A. The criminal career paradigm. In: Tonry M, Morris N, eds. *Crime and Justice: A Review of Research.* Chicago, IL: University of Chicago Press; 2003: 359–506.

53. Hahn R, McGowan A, Liberman A, et al. Effects on violence of laws and policies facilitating the transfer of youth from the juvenile to the adult justice system: a report on recommendations of the Task Force on Community Preventive Services. *MMWR Recomm Rep.* 2007; 56 (RR-9): 1–11.

54. Bishop D, Frazier C. The consequences of transfer. In: Fagan J, Zimring F, eds. *The Changing Borders of Juvenile Justice.* Chicago, IL: University of Chicago Press; 2000: 227–277.

55. Fagan J. The comparative advantage of juvenile versus criminal court sanctions on recidivism among adolescent felony offenders. *Law Policy Review.* 1996; 18: 77–119.

56. Teplin LA, Abram KM, McClelland GM, Dulcan MK, Mericle AA. Psychiatric disorders in youth in juvenile detention. *Arch Gen Psychiat.* 2002; 59(12): 1133–1143.

57. Lipsey MW. What do we learn from 400 research studies on the effectiveness of treatment with juvenile delinquents? In: McGuire J, ed. *What Works? Reducing Reoffending.* New York: John Wiley; 1995: 63–78.

58. Lipsey MW, Wilson DB, Cothern L. *Effective Intervention for Serious Juvenile Offenders.* Washington, DC: U.S. Department of Justice, Office of Juvenile Justice and Delinquency Prevention; 2000.

59. Schaeffer CM, Borduin CM. Long-term follow-up to a randomized clinical trial of multisystemic therapy with serious and violent juvenile offenders. *J Consult Clin Psych.* 2005; 73(3): 445–453.

CHAPTER 3

Child Sexual Abuse Investigations: What Every Expert Witness Needs to Know

JULIA CURCIO-ALEXANDER, JACQUELINE BLOCK
GOLDSTEIN, AND KENNETH J. WEISS

Investigations of sex crimes against children present challenges related not only to the nature of sex crimes themselves, but due to the socioemotional and cognitive characteristics of child victims. The absence of eyewitnesses and medical evidence, the belief that children are not credible witnesses, and skepticism based on concerns that children may have been exposed to suggestive interviewing, coaching, and other sources of taint create perceived barriers to obtaining reliable testimony. Child development research on children's memory and suggestibility has been used by expert witnesses as the basis of a more critical, systematic analysis of children's testimony, but not all experimental findings, or even research using convenience samples of child victims, can be generalized. Expert witness testimony on child sexual abuse accommodation syndrome (CSAAS)[1] and research on characteristics of children's disclosure have been admitted in many jurisdictions, but they have also been subjected to evidentiary challenges and limited by case law. Efforts to reduce the likelihood of suggestion and the impact of multiple interviews on children's testimony have also resulted in the use of structured child forensic interviewing protocols. The public, however, is largely unaware of the impact of these developments on investigations of sex crimes against children. Accordingly, expert witnesses in cases of alleged child sexual abuse and criminal assault must integrate a broad range of research findings, developments in investigations of crimes against children, case law, and the facts of the case in order to present information that is educative, ethical, and nonprejudicial. The purpose of this chapter is to provide an overview of information needed by expert witnesses in child sexual abuse and criminal assault cases, including the admissibility of CSAAS, relevant research, and best practices in child forensic interviewing.

The identification and prosecution of sex offenders can be frustrated when the child victim cannot cooperate due to psychological and social dynamics. Understanding CSAAS, the controversy surrounding its use in testimony, and its admissibility in court are essential for expert witnesses assisting in both defense and prosecution of alleged offenders. Summit's discussion helped to explain relational factors that influence children's responses to sexual abuse and what at first glance appear to be inexplicable behaviors.[1] While widely accepted and admissible to explain victims' behavior, the syndrome has been highly criticized due to its misuse to diagnose child sexual abuse.[2] The following sections will describe the syndrome as an interaction of child-level and environmental factors, note limits to its admissibility, and review the literature on how children disclose sexual abuse.

CHILD SEXUAL ABUSE ACCOMMODATION SYNDROME

CSAAS is a stage-based model of disclosure that was introduced into the professional literature by Summit[1] in 1983 to describe behaviors reported among sexually abused children. The model explained reasons many children do not immediately report their alleged abuse and how children's efforts to cope, particularly when alleged offenders are known to or are members of the child's family, may be misinterpreted. Summit further noted that, when children alleged sexual abuse, law enforcement, child welfare practitioners, and the courts often made determinations about the credibility of child witnesses without sufficient empirical guidance, leading to failures to protect children from individuals who had inflicted sexual trauma or to convictions of individuals who were later exonerated. CSAAS, as an empirically derived description of behavior based on clinical cases, has been widely accepted as providing valid insights into the behavioral responses of child victims of sexual abuse. As we will see later, however, it must not be used to identify a perpetrator; that is the province of the jury.

Summit's schema identifies five characteristics of child sexual abuse: (1) secrecy, (2) helplessness, (3) entrapment and accommodation, (4) delayed, conflicted, and unconvincing disclosure, and (5) retraction. *Secrecy* is described as a precondition of child sexual abuse. Child sexual abuse is typically initiated when perpetrators are alone with their victims, and eyewitnesses to these offenses are uncommon. *Helplessness* refers to the imbalance of power characteristic of perpetrator–victim relationships. Child sexual abuse most commonly occurs in the context of a relationship between the child victim and an adult or otherwise more sophisticated person. Perpetrators are often trusted family or community members, have influence on important persons in children's lives, or have the power to make decisions affecting their victims.

Secrecy and helplessness are in many cases enforced through explicit threats of harm to children and loved ones, including pets, but Summit also points out that the loss of family support may be threatening enough to ensure children's silence.[1] That is, children are dependent on caregivers for survival, and any threat of loss of those caregiving relationships or satisfaction of material and relational needs may provoke sufficient anxiety to ensure continued secrecy.[3] Power assertion in childrearing is also a factor in the expectation that children will comply with adult demands.[4] Children may also misattribute responsibility for perpetrators' behavior, internalize blame, and paradoxically seek comfort and reassurance from perpetrators.[3] Children exposed to traumatic events such as sexual abuse are at elevated risk of mood and anxiety symptoms; disruptive behavior; problems with executive functioning, including regulation of attention; substance abuse; and parasuicidal behaviors. These are problems that may further challenge children's capacity to cope but also reinforce a negative self-concept and contribute to impressions of noncredibility.[5-7] Further, the impact of sexual abuse coupled with the impact of living with "anticipatory dread" of subsequent assaults may precipitate internalized efforts to escape such as denial, dissociation, and other efforts to detach from overwhelming emotions.[8] These child-level and relational factors interact to compel children's accommodation of sexual abuse.

· On the surface, the complexity of relational and other factors among child victims, perpetrators, and nonoffending caregivers may create a confusing picture for investigators and others. However, a closer look may clarify Summit's next three CSAAS characteristics: *entrapment and accommodation, delayed disclosure*, and *retracting allegations*. Entrapment and accommodation occur when child victims are unable to break through the many relational and situational barriers to overcoming the secrecy surrounding their abuse and are subjected to continued abuse and in many cases increasingly intrusive, frightening, and painful assaults.[1] The secrecy of child sexual abuse, children's experiences of coercion, misattribution of responsibility, and the increased risk of psychopathology are understood to be factors in delayed disclosure, unwillingness to disclose, and retracting allegations. Lack of medical evidence and of eyewitnesses or other corroboration leads criminal and child welfare investigators to depend entirely on appraisals of victim credibility.[9-11] Young children and those with cognitive and language delays may have limited ability to understand and express the nature of their abusive experiences. These limitations, in additional to the relational factors outlined above that may underlie delayed, incremental, or retracted disclosures, are often the reasons adults may view child witnesses as relatively less credible and result in "unfounded report" determinations by child welfare authorities and decisions by law enforcement and prosecutors to not pursue criminal charges.

Presentations of CSAAS by expert witnesses typically highlight children's accommodation to sexual assault in an effort to help civil and criminal courts make sense of seemingly counterintuitive victim behavior. CSAAS as a child-level syndrome, however, results from an interaction of children's characteristics and those of various levels of children's ecologies, including family, community, healthcare providers, schools, law enforcement, and courts. The ecological/transactional view holds that child-level characteristics and the environment operate in a mutually interactive way to affect children's outcomes.[12,13] Areas of research influenced by the ecological/transactional model include studies of child maltreatment and onset of psychopathology, and the impact of domestic violence on children's development.[14,15] From this perspective, it becomes equally important to examine both the impact of children's abusive experiences on their disclosures and perceived credibility and also the role of caregivers, healthcare practitioners, law enforcement, and court systems in maintaining the secrecy of sexual abuse, children's helplessness, entrapment and accommodation, and difficulties disclosing. Striking case examples of this interplay of environment and child-level characteristics in recent media include the highly publicized criminal prosecutions of Gerald Sandusky and the Monsignor William Lynn in Pennsylvania. These cases illustrate key features of the CSAAS pattern as an interaction of children and multiple levels of their ecologies (e.g., family, community, law enforcement). These cases have provided strong empirical support for Summit's construct.

However, acceptance of the CSAAS schema has not been unequivocal.[16] Summit himself criticized misuse of the syndrome and reiterated that CSAAS is a "clinical observation" and not diagnostic or proof of sexual abuse.[17] Despite this clarification, many jurisdictions continued to struggle with the implication that the presence of behaviors characteristic of CSAAS may lead the courts and child welfare authorities to conclude that children's allegations are valid. While helpful to prosecutors, misuse of CSAAS in testimony may have had a role in some wrongful convictions. Historical misapplication in use of the construct, concern that admission of syndromal evidence could bias juries against the accused, and subsequent research suggesting that not all features of CSAAS are present in all cases combine to strongly suggest that experts may make clearer presentations by referencing the research on children's disclosures rather than arguing the presence or absence of a syndrome. The next section will present an overview of children's disclosure research.

Since Summit introduced and later clarified the use of CSAAS, a considerable body of research has emerged examining in more detail characteristics of children's disclosures of sexual abuse. The child sexual abuse research literature is unequivocal in its support of Summit's position that child victims often delay disclosure or do not disclose at all during childhood. London and colleagues[18] examined 13 retrospective studies and found that 55% to 69% of adult survivors of child sexual abuse said that they did not disclose the abuse at all during childhood. A second finding of their review was that only 5% to 13%, across studies of participants, reported sexual abuse to authorities during childhood.[18] An early study by Finkelhor and colleagues[19] found that 27% of the women and 16% of the men in their national survey reported histories of child sexual abuse; of these, 42% disclosed the abuse within 1 year, 20% disclosed it later than 1 year, and 38% never disclosed the abuse until their participation in the survey.

Research also supports the position that children who disclose may produce inconsistent, unconvincing statements. One small study included forensic interviews of 10 children who were sexually assaulted by a common perpetrator who had videotaped 102 of the assaults.[20] The children had made no disclosures prior to the interviews. The researchers rated the severity of the videotaped sexual abuse and victim interviews. The severity ratings of the children's descriptions of abuse during interviews were significantly lower than the ratings of the victims' videotaped sexual abuse, and none of the children reported abuse that was inconsistent with the video content. That is, the children in this study who were confirmed victims of sexual assault significantly minimized and denied sexual abuse. In another study of 21 children who tested positive for gonorrhea, only 43% alleged sexual abuse.[21]

Nondisclosure has also been studied under controlled conditions. A 1991 study of nonabused children corroborated the above findings.[22] Seventy-five nonabused girls between the ages of 5 and 7 were given physical examinations for scoliosis under one of two conditions. In one group the physical examination included genital and anal touching (genital condition). The second group's physical examination excluded genital and anal touching (nongenital condition). During interviews, 78% of the children in the genital condition failed to reveal vaginal touching and 89% failed to reveal anal touching. When asked direct questions with anatomically detailed dolls, 14% failed to disclose genital touching and 21% failed to disclose anal touching. Of particular interest, none of the children in the nongenital condition falsely reported genital touch in response to free recall or the doll demonstration. When the children were asked direct questions, the false report rate was 3% for genital touching and 6% for anal touching. These results indicate that direct questions may elicit more valid responses from children who have experienced genital and anal touching. Of the 3% who falsely disclosed genital touching, two thirds could not elaborate.[22] Overall, research provides confirming data that are not commonly available in child sexual abuse investigations and offers compelling support for the position that children minimize and deny abuse.

The research on recanting is more difficult to interpret. In London and colleagues' review, the authors noted only a 4% to 27% rate of recanted allegations in *confirmed* cases of sexual abuse.[18] The assumption that the rate of confirmed abuse cases is a reliable proxy for the number of true abuse cases is likely to be invalid, as a recanted allegation is a common reason for unsubstantiated reports. Research confirms that many children who have experienced abuse at some point recant their statements. Following disclosure and during investigation, children's fears about disclosure may become a reality and precipitate retracting in an effort to restore ruptured family and community relationships. Children commonly recant allegations in response to pressure from family members during investigations, and prosecutors often call on experts to provide testimony on CSAAS to rehabilitate the child's testimony.[23,24]

Child-level factors and characteristics of children's ecologies have been associated with disclosure in other studies. Males are less likely to disclose due to concerns with being identified as homosexual (when the perpetrator is male) and the belief that males cannot be victims.[25-27] Children who are relatively older at the time of a forensic interview are more likely to disclose compared to younger children, in part due to language development and other cognitive differences.[20,27] Family-level characteristics are also related to children's disclosures. Retrospective studies of adults who were sexually abused as children by a parent or parent figure find lower rates of disclosure compared to children who were abused by someone outside of the family.[18,28] Fear of retaliation, including physical harm; rejection by loved ones, including nonoffending caregivers; and concerns that the perpetrator would be incarcerated were related in other studies to lower levels of disclosure.[27,29] Similarly, recanting allegations was found to be more likely when the child was sexually abused by a family member, when the nonoffending caregiver was unsupportive, and when the victim was younger than 10 years.[28]

INDIVIDUAL DIFFERENCES

Experts need to consider individual differences and the influence of environment on children's capacity to recall and describe their experiences. Several child-level and environmental factors are related to children's cognitive and socioemotional development. The quality and quantity of spoken language in the home are related to children's cognitive development, varying also with maternal education and socioeconomic status.[30-32] Young children growing up in poverty are more than twice as likely to have cognitive delays and to experience poorer physical and emotional health and behavioral problems.[33,34] A number of studies have found relationships between children's language acquisition and maternal talkativeness, maternal depression, size of maternal vocabulary, maternal syntactic complexity and maternal responsiveness.[30] Nelson and Fivush[35] noted that children's developing language and narrative skills are developed through participation in dialogue with caregivers about past experiences. These exchanges facilitate children's evolving understanding of past and present time. Given the relationship of poverty to a range of problems, including the potential for compromised cognitive development, experts are recommended to keep in mind the impact of multiple risk exposures on children's capacity to describe their experiences.

TESTIMONY ON CHILDREN'S MEMORY AND SUGGESTIBILITY

Expert witnesses in child sexual abuse and criminal assault cases need to be knowledgeable about childhood memory development in order to evaluate interviews and testimony. Studies of memory development often distinguish between implicit or nondeclarative memory and declarative memory, which emerges with language acquisition and is verbally mediated.[36,37] One of the defining characteristics of nondeclarative or implicit memory is that it is not consciously accessible but can exert effects on cognition, emotion, and behavior. Conditioning experiments with infants as young as 3 months confirm that babies can remember both objects and their behavior with those objects.[38] The impact of nondeclarative memory on the behavior of sexually abused young children may include developmentally atypical sexual behaviors. These young children, while unable to use words to describe their experiences, may express their experiences through repetitive reenacting of abusive events. These behaviors, while clinically relevant, are unlikely to stand on their own as evidence and need to be considered along with other case information.

Children's ability to provide verbal testimony emerges with the development of language and declarative memory. Declarative memory is verbally mediated and consists of two subsystems. *Semantic memory* contains general information about the world that is represented through language (e.g., knowing that Canada lies north of the United States). *Episodic memory,* also known as autobiographical memory, is defined as memory for personally experienced events, including location, time of event, and associated sensations and emotions (e.g., the experience of visiting Canada).[39] Episodic memory develops between the ages of 4 and 7 years, with progressive gains in the capacity to recall and describe experienced events.[40] This trajectory accounts for differences between preschool and school-aged children's responses to open-ended, free-recall questions during investigative interviews, with school-aged children providing more detailed responses.

Children are less likely to remember and describe events for which they have no frame of reference for interpreting and understanding.[41] In addition to limited development of episodic memory, preschoolers also do not have well-developed memory retrieval strategies compared to older children. Overall, the research consistently demonstrates that children's descriptions of experienced events become more detailed and accurate as a function of age and cognitive development.[42,43] One caveat is that school-aged children are more likely to remember the details of the content of experienced events over the timing of events.[44,45] That is, children may be more likely to report accurately about *what* occurred compared to *when* it occurred.

Expert witnesses are often called upon to testify on empirical findings about factors related to the accuracy of children's reports of their experiences. In these cases, experts do not interview or clinically evaluate witnesses but educate triers of fact on scientific findings relevant to questions of children's reliability as witnesses. Experts may also offer an opinion on the extent to which a particular investigation adhered to recommended professional guidelines.[46] Research has established that children are often capable of reporting accurately about their experiences.[47]

An influential line of investigation into declarative memory finds that retrieval is based on reconstruction of fragments rather than location of a replica.[48] This characteristic of memory retrieval makes the veracity of memories highly vulnerable to suggestion. Many studies have established that under particular sets of laboratory conditions, significant proportions of both children and adults will report memories of entirely false events, providing details and even expressing emotions congruent with false memories.[49,50] Contrary to popular opinion, however, children may not be at increased risk of suggestion relative to adults. Several recent studies have contradicted a sizable body of research previously finding age declines in false memory and suggestibility.[51,52] On the contrary, these studies have found that accuracy declined and false memories increased with age due to an increase in gist- and meaning-driven rather than verbatim reconstruction.[53] What these findings suggest in practical terms is that a preference for semantic memory extracted from repeated experiences of a similar type (i.e., gist traces), as opposed to memories of detailed verbatim representations, is related to increases in false memories with age.

As informative as these finding are, their ecological validity may be limited. Suggestibility concerns during investigations of child abuse are due to questions about whether children were coached to deny abuse that actually occurred or to allege abuse that did not occur or were inadvertently influenced by caregivers or investigators. Instances of children being coached to falsely allege abuse is considered to represent proportionally few cases relative to all reports of abuse. The more common situation is coaching of children by offending and nonoffending caregivers to conceal or retract valid allegations of abuse.[54,55] Another source of taint—innocuous influences exerted by investigators and caregivers—may include caregiver conversations about experienced abuse and concerns about potentially leading interview questions. As we will note in the sections to follow, interviewer sources of taint have been systematically addressed through the use of empirically validated investigative interview protocols and the use of Child Advocacy Centers to eliminate repeat interviews and interviews by untrained investigators.

FORENSIC INTERVIEWING WITH CHILDREN: EVIDENCE BASE FOR TESTIMONY

Children who are alleged to have been sexually abused are referred in many jurisdictions for a forensic interview during investigation. The purpose of a forensic interview is to obtain a thorough and accurate description of the alleged maltreatment or offense, to determine if a child is likely to have been a victim of maltreatment or a crime, and, if possible, to identify the alleged perpetrator. Decisions based on forensic interview data, together with physical examination and laboratory evidence, include criminal charging decisions by law enforcement and whether to substantiate reports of child maltreatment by child protective services. Forensic interview data may also inform evaluation and treatment recommendations, including medical and behavioral health assessments. Several forensic interviewing protocols are currently in use. Some of the most commonly used are the Step Wise Interview,[56] the National Institute of Child Health and Development (NICHD) Investigative Interview Protocol,[57] and the National Child Advocacy Center (CAC) model.[58] Characteristics common to structured interview protocols developed for use with child witnesses include an initial phase of rapport building, practice interviews on neutral topics, establishing that children understand the difference between the truth and falsehood or fantasy, and instructing the child to report accurately with no guessing. The Step Wise Interview is an early investigative interview protocol that provided guidelines for the use of open-ended questions and the importance of keeping several hypotheses in mind about the range of possible experiences and events that may have led to the allegations. These guidelines minimize suggestive interview questions and the likelihood of interviewer bias and of the interviewer communicating knowledge of the allegations to an interviewee.

The NICHD Investigative Interview Protocol is the most widely researched of all the structured forensic interview protocols. This research grew out of a broader study of children's capacity to remember and describe their experiences accurately, and under what conditions children may be more or less suggestible. Based upon this research, a consensus emerged regarding best practices for use of forensic interviews with child witnesses, including the need to establish rapport, provide episodic memory training by interviewing the child on a neutral topic, assess whether the child understands the difference between truth and a lie, and provide ground rules (e.g., instructions to provide factual information only) and the use of open-ended questions, with follow-up questions, including option-posing questions and cued-recognition prompts, near the end of the interview when needed to gather more details about reported events.[47]

Field studies have established that the NICHD protocol, compared to traditional interview protocols, has utility in gathering forensically relevant information in a manner that minimizes the need for recognition probes. In one study, two groups of alleged victims of child sexual abuse were matched on age, perpetrator relationship, and severity of abuse.[59] One group participated in a traditional interview protocol, the other in the NICHD protocol. Of the children in the NICHD group, 89% disclosed sexual abuse in response to open-ended questions only. Only 36% of the children participating in traditional protocols disclosed. Other studies have demonstrated that NICHD interviews, compared to traditional interviews, contain a higher proportion of open-ended questions overall and a higher number of open-ended questions occurring before the introduction of option-posing questions. These findings are critical to decisions about the validity of interview findings, as studies have consistently found that open-ended questions and free recall produce more accurate responses.[59-62] Studies examining the relationship of NICHD interview variables and case outcomes found that criminal charges were more likely to be filed after use of the NICHD protocol compared to non-protocol interviews and were more likely to result in a guilty plea.[63]

As noted, the NICHD protocol is the most widely researched of the investigative interview protocols, but the structured interviews currently used during investigations of child maltreatment and crimes against children have identical well-researched components (e.g., rapport building, truth–lie discussions, introduction to ground rules, practice interviews, use of open-ended questions). The CAC protocol, however, takes the procedure even further. In addition to using a structured forensic interview protocol, the CAC model has a multidisciplinary approach that minimizes the number of interviews and interviewers. Interviews take place in a safe, supportive, child-friendly setting. A highly trained and well-supervised forensic interviewer conducts the structured interview, but other parties who require interview data participate by concurrently observing the interview (e.g., through a one-way mirror) and are provided with opportunities to consult with the lead interviewer and suggest additional questions. Forensic interviewers receive training at the National Child Advocacy Center in Huntsville, Alabama, or at trainings provided regionally by national or local CAC staff. Other participants typically include law enforcement, child protective services, and prosecutors. The CAC protocol was developed in response to concerns about the unreliability of children's testimony when participating in multiple interviews conducted by individuals without training in child development and forensic interviewing. Reforms endorsed by professional practice organizations, including the American Professional Society on the Abuse of Children, incorporate standardized training and practice guidelines at over 700 CAC sites nationwide.[58,64]

Regardless of the choice of protocol, expert witnesses providing testimony on forensic interviews must be able to explain the components of the protocol used and whether the interviewer adhered to the protocol to the maximum extent possible given the child and the circumstances. If modifications were made, the expert will need to determine if those modifications were the result of deliberate decision making that can be explained. For example, an interviewer may elect to use aids such as allowing the child to draw or use an anatomically detailed doll to encourage greater responsiveness and accuracy during interviews when the child's motivation, language development, or other cognitive limitations are an issue.[65] Further, expert witnesses need to be knowledgeable about the range of forensic interview protocols in use, including their similarities and differences. For the most part, existing protocols are more similar than they are different. The primary distinction is the use of interview aids and whether they are routinely used to assess children's knowledge of their body parts and provide visual cues to help children retrieve details.

Regardless of which forensic interviewing protocol is being used, there is consensus that the use of open-ended questions that elicit narrative responses is preferred, thus minimizing suggestiveness and increasing the accuracy of children's statements.[46] Research has confirmed that most children will disclose in response to open-ended questions that contain no references to allegations of abuse.[66] Interviewers are encouraged to use a "funnel technique" whereby questions remain open-ended and become more focused and direct only later in the interview.[67] Open-ended and free-recall questions are often too vague to help younger children and those who have less sophisticated language and retrieval strategies become oriented to the purpose of the interview and responses needed. After forensically relevant details have been obtained, the interviewer reverts to open-ended follow-up questions to gain more free-recall information. While multiple-choice questions are inherently more suggestive than open-ended questions because they provide content options, the presence of a nonspecific, open-ended option helps to keep the question from becoming forced choice.[68] It should be noted that CAC interviewers, guided by best practice standards, would not confirm sexual abuse based on a *yes* response and no further elaboration. Additional standards suggest that interviewers avoid repeating questions that the child has already answered, avoid asking a reticent child to imagine what might have happened or introducing material the child has not already disclosed, and avoid letting the child know that the interviewer is aware that allegations were reported and are under investigation.[59]

LIMITS ON TESTIMONY

An understanding of research on children's disclosures of sexual abuse, memory development, and investigative interview protocols is critical for expert witnesses, but experts need to be mindful of the extent to which research findings can be generalized. *External validity* concerns questions of whether the findings of research studies can be generalized to individuals who did not participate in the study. A closely related term is *ecological validity*, in which the question concerns whether study findings can be generalized to settings other than the one in which the study was conducted.[69] For example, laboratory studies of implanted memories using child participants may not be generalizable to children being coached by caregivers to falsely allege, deny, or retract abuse allegations since the relational context and other situational variables would not be comparable. To overgeneralize research findings to discredit a child witness is ethically suspect. Case law sets constraints on testimony in that it may not be used to imply that an alleged perpetrator is responsible for the abuse or guilty of an offense.[70,71] There are as yet no published examples of case law that applies the same principle and constrains testimony intended to discredit victims, so the expert needs to be knowledgeable about the studies used. The expert witness is advised to maintain a neutral stance and provide valid and helpful information to child protective services, law enforcement, and the courts.

REFERENCES

1. Summit RC. The child sexual abuse accommodation syndrome. *Child Abuse Neglect*. 1983; 7: 177–193.
2. Weiss KJ, Alexander JC. Sex, lies and statistics: inferences from the child sexual abuse accommodation syndrome. *J Am Acad Psychiatry Law*. 2013; 41: 412–420.
3. Prior S. *Object Relations in Severe Trauma: Psychotherapy of the Sexually Abused Child*. Lanham, MD: Rowman & Littlefield; 1996.
4. Baumrind D. Differentiating between confrontive and coercive kinds of parental power assertive disciplinary practices. *Human Development*. 2012; 55: 35–51.

5. Shiu M. Unwarranted skepticism: the federal courts' treatment of child sexual abuse accommodation syndrome. *Southern California Interdisciplinary Law Journal*. 2009; 18: 651–677.

6. Quas J, Goodman G, Bidrose S, Pipe M, Craw S, Ablin D. Emotion and memory: children's long-term remembering, forgetting, and suggestibility. *J Exp Child Psychol*. 1999; 72: 235–270.

7. Beers SR, DeBellis MD. Neuropsychological function in children with maltreatment-related posttraumatic stress disorder. *Am J Psychiatry*. 2002; 159: 483–486.

8. Terr LC. Childhood traumas: An outline and overview. *Am J Psychiatry*. 1991; 148: 10–20.

9. Heger A, Ticson L, Velasquez O, Bernier, R. Children referred for possible sexual abuse: medical findings in 2384 children. *Child Abuse Neglect*. 2002; 26: 645–659.

10. Everson ED, Sandoval JM, Bernson N, Crowson M, Robinson H. Reliability of professional judgments in forensic child sexual abuse evaluations: unsettled or unsettling science? *J Child Sex Abuse*. 2012; 21: 72–90.

11. Walsh WA, Cross TP, Jones LM, Simone M, Kolko DJ. Which sexual abuse victims receive a forensic medical examination? The impact of Children's Advocacy Centers. *Child Abuse Neglect*. 2007; 31: 1053–1068.

12. Bronfenbrenner U. *The Ecology of Human Development: Experiments by Nature and Design*. Cambridge, MA: Harvard University Press; 1979.

13. Sameroff AJ, Chandler MJ. Reproductive risk and the continuum of caretaking casualty. In: Horowitz FD, Hetherington M, Scarr-Salapatek S, Siegel G, eds. *Review of Child Development Research*, vol. 4. Chicago: University of Chicago Press; 1975: 187–244.

14. Cicchetti D, Toth SL. A developmental psychopathology perspective on child abuse and neglect. *J Am Acad Child Adolesc Psychiatry*. 1995; 34: 541–565.

15. Fantuzzo J, Perlman S. The unique impact of out-of-home placement and the mediating effects of child maltreatment and homelessness on early school success. *Youth Services Review*. 2007; 29: 941–960.

16. Ceci SJ, Bruck M. *Jeopardy in the Courtroom: A Scientific Analysis of Children's Testimony*. Washington, DC: American Psychological Association; 1995.

17. Summit R. Abuse of the child sexual abuse accommodation syndrome. *J Child Sex Abus*. 1992; 1: 153–163.

18. London K, Bruck M, Wright DB, Ceci SJ. Review of the contemporary literature on how children report sexual abuse to others: findings, methodological issues, and implications for forensic interviewers. *Memory*. 2008; 16: 29–47.

19. Finkelhor D, Hotaling G, Lewis IA, Smith C. Sexual abuse in a national survey of adult men and women: prevalence, characteristics, and risk factors. *Child Abuse Neglect*. 1990; 14: 19–28.

20. Sjoberg RL, Lindblad F. Limited disclosure of sexual abuse in children whose experiences were documented by videotape. *Am J Psychiatry*. 2002; 159: 312–314.

21. Lyon TD. False denials: overcoming methodological biases in abuse disclosure research. In: Pipe ME, Lamb ME, Orbach Y, Cederborg AC, eds. *Disclosing Abuse: Delays, Denials, Retractions and Incomplete Accounts*. Mahwah, NJ: Erlbaum; 2007: 41–62.

22. Saywitz K, Goodman G, Nicholas G, Moan S. Children's memory of a physical examination involving genital touch: implications for reports of child sexual abuse. *J Consul Clin Psychol.* 1991; 5: 682–691.
23. Paine MI, Hanson DJ. Factors influencing children to self-disclose sexual abuse. *Clin Psychol Rev.* 2002; 22: 271–295.
24. Sorenson T, Snow B. How children tell: the process of disclosure in child sexual abuse. *Child Welfare.* 1991; 70: 3–15.
25. Alaggia R. Disclosing the trauma of child sexual abuse: a gender analysis. *J Loss Trauma.* 2005; 10: 453–470.
26. Ghetti S, Goodman GS, Eisen ML, Qin J, Davis SL. Consistency in children's reports of sexual and physical abuse. *Child Abuse Neglect.* 2002; 26: 977–995.
27. Lippert T, Cross TP, Jones L, Walsh W. Telling interviewers about sexual abuse: predictors of child disclosure at forensic interviews. *Child Maltreatment.* 2009; 14: 100–113.
28. Malloy LC, Lyon TD, Quas JA. Filial dependency and recantation of child sexual abuse allegations. *J Am Acad Child Adolesc Psychiatry.* 2007; 46: 162–170.
29. Malloy LC, Brubacher SP, Lamb ME. Expected consequences of disclosure revealed in investigative interviews with suspected victims of child sexual abuse. *Appl Dev Sci.* 2011; 15: 8–19.
30. Eigsti MI, Cicchetti D. The impact of child maltreatment on expressive syntax at 60 months. *Dev Sci.* 2004; 7: 88–102.
31. Hart B, Risley TR. *Meaningful Differences in the Everyday Experience of Young American Children.* Baltimore, MD: Brookes Publishing; 1995.
32. Hoff E. The specificity of environmental influence: socioeconomic status affects early vocabulary development via maternal speech. *Child Development.* 2003; 74: 1368–1378.
33. Bradle RH, Corwyn RF. Socioeconomic status and child development. *Annu Rev Psychol.* 2002; 5: 371–399.
34. Leventhal T, Brooks-Gunn J. The neighborhoods they live in: the effects of neighborhood residence on child and adolescent outcomes. *Psychol Bull.* 2002; 126: 309–337.
35. Nelson K, Fivush R. The emergence of autobiographical memory: a social cultural developmental theory. *Psychol Rev.* 2004; 111: 486–511.
36. Lieberman AF. Traumatic stress and quality of attachment: reality and internalization in disorders of infant mental health. *Infant Ment Health J.* 2004; 25: 336–351.
37. Scheeringa MS, Gaenbauer TJ. Posttraumatic stress disorder. In: Zeanah CH Jr., ed. *Handbook of Infant Mental Health.* 2nd ed. New York: Guildford Press; 1999: 369–381.
38. Gerhardstein P, Liu J, Rovee-Collier C. Perceptual constraints on infant memory retrieval. *J Exp Child Psychol.* 1998; 69: 109–131.
39. Tulving E. Episodic memory: from mind to brain. *Annu Rev Psychol.* 2002; 53: 1–25.
40. Yim H, Dennis SJ, Sloutsky VM. The development of episodic memory: items, contexts, and relations. *Psychol Sci.* 2013; 24: 2163–2172.
41. Ornstein PA, Shapiro LR, Clubb PA, Follmer A, Baker-Ward L. The influence of prior knowledge on children's memory for salient medical experiences. In: Stein NL, Ornstein PA, Brainerd CJ, Tversky B, eds. *Memory for Everyday and Emotional Events.* Hillsdale, NJ: Erlbaum; 1997: 83–111.

42. Brainerd CJ. The reliability of children's testimony. *Child and Adolescent Behavior Newsletter.* 1994.

43. Pipe ME, Sutherland R, Webster N, Jones C, La Rooy D. Do early interviews affect children's long-term event recall? *Appl Cog Psychol.* 2004; 18: 823–839.

44. Friedman WJ, Reese E, Dai X. Children's memory for the times of events from the past years. *Appl Cog Psychol.* 2010; 25: 156–165.

45. Pathman T, Burch M, Bauer MM. Young children's memory for the times of personal past events. *J Cogn Dev.* 2013; 14: 120–140.

46. Buck JA, London K, Wright DB. Expert testimony regarding child witnesses: does it sensitize jurors to forensic interview quality? *Law Hum Behav.* 2011; 35: 152–164.

47. Lamb ME, Orbach Y, Hershkowitz I, Esplin P, Horowitz D. A structured interview protocol improves the quality and informativeness of investigative interviews with children: a review of research using the NICHD Investigative Interview Protocol. *Child Abuse Neglect.* 2007; 21: 1201–1231.

48. Stark C, Okado Y, Loftus EF. Imaging the reconstruction of true and false memories using sensory reactivation and the misinformation paradigms. *Learn Mem.* 2010; 17: 485–488.

49. Ceci SJ, Huffman MLC, Smith E, Loftus EF. Repeatedly thinking about non-events. *Conscious Cogn.* 1994; 3: 388–407.

50. Loftus EF. Creating false memories. *Sci Am.* 1997; 277: 70–75.

51. Chae Y, Ceci SJ. Individual differences in children's recall and suggestibility: the effect of intelligence, temperament, and self-perceptions. *Appl Cog Psychol.* 2005; 19: 383–407.

52. Young K, Powell MB, Dudgeon P. Individual differences in children's suggestibility: a comparison between intellectually disabled and mainstream samples. *Pers Indiv Dif.* 2003; 1: 31–49.

53. Brainerd CJ, Reyna VF. Fuzzy-trace theory and children's false memories. *J Exp Child Psychol.* 1998; 71: 81–129.

54. Faller KC. *Maltreatment in Early Childhood: Tools for Research-Based Intervention.* Binghamton, NY: Haworth Press; 1999.

55. Leichtman MD, Ceci SJ. The effects of stereotypes and suggestions on preschoolers reports. *Dev Psychol.* 1995; 31: 568–578.

56. Yuille JC, Hunter R, Joffe R, Zaparniuk J. Interviewing children in sexual abuse cases. In: Goodman GS, Bottoms GL, eds. *Child Victims, Child Witnesses: Understanding and Improving Children's Testimony.* New York: Guilford Press; 1993: 95–115.

57. Sternberg KJ, Lamb ME, Esplin PW, Orbach Y, Hershkowitz I. Using a structured interview protocol to improve the quality of investigative interviews. In: Eisen ML, Quas JA, Goodman ES, eds. *Memory and Suggestibility in the Forensic Interview.* Mahwah, NJ: Erlbaum; 2002: 409–436.

58. Cross T, Jones L, Walsh W, et al. Evaluating Children's Advocacy Centers' response to child sexual abusey. Juvenile Justice Bulletin. 2008: Office of Juvenile Justice and Delinquency Prevention, U.S. Department of Justice. Retrieved January 2, 2014, from http://www.ncjrs.gov/pdffiles1/ojjdp/218530.pdf

59. Sternberg KJ, Lamb ME, Orbach Y, Esplin PW, Mitchell S. Use of a structured investigative protocol enhances young children's responses to free recall prompts in the course of forensic interviews. *J Appl Psychol.* 2001; 85: 997–1005.

60. Ceci SJ, Loftus EF, Leichtman M, Bruck M. The role of source misattributions in the creation of false beliefs among pre-schoolers. *Int J Clin Exp Hypn*. 1994; 62: 304–320.

61. Lamb ME, Sternberg KJ, Orbach Y, Esplin PW, Stewart H, Mitchell S. Age differences in young children's responses to open-ended invitations in the course of forensic interviews. *J Consult Clin Psychol*. 2003; 71: 926–934.

62. Loftus EF. Leading questions and the eyewitness report. *Cogn Psychol*. 1974; 7: 560–572.

63. Pipe M, Orbach Y, Lamb M, Abbott CB, Stewart H. Do best practice interviews with child abuse victims influence case processing? Research report submitted to the U.S. Department of Justice; 2008. Retrieved January 2, 2014, from http://www.ncjrs.gov/pdffiles1/nij/grants/224524.pdf

64. Jones LM, Cross TP, Walsh WA, Simone M. Criminal investigations of child abuse: the research behind "best practices." *Trauma Violence Abuse*. 2005; 6: 254–268.

65. Everson MD, Boat BW. The utility of anatomical dolls and drawings in child forensic interviews. In: Eisen ML, Quas JA, Goodman GS, eds. *Memory and Suggestibility in the Forensic Interview*. Mahwah, NJ: Erlbaum; 2002: 383–408.

66. Perona A, Bottoms B, Sorenson E. Research-based guidelines for child forensic interviews. In: *Ending Child Abuse: New Efforts in Prevention, Investigation, and Training*. New York: Haworth Press; 2006.

67. Yuille JC, Cutshall JL. A case study of eyewitness memory of a crime. *J Appl Psychol*. 1986; 71: 291–301.

68. Poole D, White L. Effects of question repetition on the eyewitness testimony of children and adults. *Dev Psychol*. 1991; 27: 975–986.

69. Dekkers OM, von Elm E, Algra A, Vandenbroucke JA. How to assess the external validity of therapeutic trials: a conceptual approach. *Int J Epidemiol*. 2010; 39: 89–94.

70. *New Jersey* v. P.H., 178 N.J. 378 (2004).

71. *New Jersey* v. *Schnabel*, 196 N.J. 116 (2008).

CHAPTER 4

Stress, Trauma, and the Developing Brain

JOHN K. NORTHROP AND STEVEN J. BERKOWITZ

The practice of forensic psychiatry requires a wide range of expertise and knowledge in order to evaluate patients and educate the court about one's findings. While often not an explicit aspect of an evaluation in a criminal or civil proceeding, a comprehensive forensic evaluation includes the individual's trauma history—for example, child abuse and neglect and their possible contributions to impairments in functioning and coping.

Relevant in correctional settings, studies have demonstrated that large percentages of both incarcerated men and women have histories of childhood maltreatment.[1] Research has demonstrated that in the majority of criminal cases, the forensic psychiatrist is working with a population whose pathology and behavioral problems are heavily rooted in the experience of chronic and cumulative adverse events or stressors in childhood.[1] Assessing for established trauma-related syndromes, such as posttraumatic stress disorder (PTSD), is standard but may not capture the range of disorders and impairments caused by childhood adversity. PTSD is only one of multiple difficulties and disorders that result from traumatic and adverse experiences in childhood and is probably not the most common.[2-7]

In this chapter we provide an overview of studies demonstrating the pernicious and lasting impact of childhood maltreatment on health and social outcomes in adulthood. Next, we outline scientific progress toward understanding the biomolecular changes that result from maltreatment and chronic stress and commonly persist into adulthood. With a developing body of evidence both in the epidemiology and neurobiology of childhood maltreatment and stress, the forensic examiner is better positioned to educate the court in criminal cases regarding the psychological damage and its biologic basis for the dysfunction. We aim to provide the forensic psychiatrist with an enriched understanding of childhood trauma and how to assess for it; how to recognize its lasting effects on neurophysiology, cognition, emotions, and behavior; and how to comment on it scientifically in the forensic report and testimony.

CHILDHOOD MALTREATMENT: BEYOND PTSD

Trauma is an ancient Greek word meaning injury or wound, adopted by the medical field to connote serious injury (e.g., trauma surgery). Psychological trauma may be understood as an experience or group of experiences causing injury to the brain, having the capacity to deregulate neurophysiology (and potentially general physiology) as well as cognitive, emotional, and behavioral functioning. As in most injuries, recovery and healing usually occur with little or no intervention. However, some injuries are more severe and require treatment to heal, while others result in permanent damage and impaired or perturbed functioning. The most insidious injuries are those caused by chronic, negatively stressful or traumatizing experiences. Importantly, the impact of these experiences varies from individual to individual, and different individuals may be resilient to or injured by the same events or set of events.

Two of the frequent misconceptions encountered, and characteristic of the lay understanding of childhood maltreatment, are derived from outmoded ideas about nature versus nurture and the dichotomization of mind and brain. While the mental health field has evolved in its understanding, most non-mental health professionals still view mental illness as either etiologically biologic and genetic (e.g., schizophrenia or autism) or a congenital injury or later-in-life physical insult (e.g., anoxia, *in utero* toxic exposure, infection, traumatic brain injury, stroke). In the lay minds of judges and jurors, trauma is often regarded as the result of adverse experiences and thus only a disorder of the mind, rather than a brain disorder with a biologic and anatomic basis. In contrast, mounting research demonstrates that life experiences interface in the brain at the molecular and structural levels over time. It is very difficult to explain in lay terms how behavior and function, and the whole individual, are affected by traumatic and adverse experience. Yet, the task of the expert witness is to bring these dynamics to life in a manner that is scientifically sound and relevant to the legal question.

It is increasingly clear that humans may best be understood as analogous to biologic "machines" in which the only possible mechanisms by which humans function are biologic, and that the mind is a primary brain function. One good example is simple learning. For a new fact or skill to be acquired, there are biomolecular changes that permit learning and memory. As Kandel[8] demonstrated in his groundbreaking laboratory research, learning means *physical* changes in the nervous system. An example is the finding that babies born with cataracts and untreated will be blind because the visual cortex requires stimuli perceived through the eyes to organize and decode visual input. *Mind* can be understood as a dynamic interplay between the brain and the outside world, so any external stimulus (i.e., experience) must affect the brain and vice versa. The notion of gene–environment interaction and epigenetic mechanisms as an explanatory model of the manner in which traumatizing experiences are biologic processes is a recent and complex concept. Helping non-mental-health professionals such as jurors and judges understand the importance and relevance of these ideas in understanding attachment, symptoms, and behavior is critical.

ADVERSE CHILDHOOD EXPERIENCES AND THEIR SIGNIFICANCE

Adverse experience is a term more commonly used in recent years as a result of the Adverse Childhood Experience (ACE) Study.[6,7] In many journal articles and the lay press, adverse experience is used synonymously with trauma. However, the ACE Study did not evaluate histories of childhood trauma. Instead, it asked about a wide range of 10 adverse experiences, from divorce to child abuse. The positive responses were summed to derive an ACE score that predicted later medical problems. In the multiple projects employing ACE Study methodology, investigators have found repeatedly that a score of 4 or more is highly correlated with psychiatric disorders and medical and behavioral issues.[9] While having been exposed to one ACE was not necessarily traumatic (i.e., injurious), it does increase the risk for poor behavioral outcomes marginally, but having 4 or more increased the risk of traumatization (i.e., injury).

Given the subtle distinction between the accumulation of adverse experience and a single traumatic incident, the confusion between an adverse experience and a traumatic experience is understandable. Having experienced 1 ACE is predictive of having experienced more ACEs, since exposures to bad experiences tend to cluster.[10,11] In addition, youth who have encountered multiple adverse experiences are likely to experience a more objectively horrifying event or classic traumatic experience.[11] To avoid this understandable confusion, we have defined an adverse experience as one that typically causes distress but may or may not cause injury that is long lasting or requires intervention, while an accumulation of adverse experience can cause trauma (i.e., injury) and changes in functioning. That is, traumatic experience, by this definition, causes an injury, while adverse experience may or may not. Perhaps a more recognizable manner of understanding the findings from the ACE studies is that the accumulation of ACEs is a proxy for chronic unremitting stress during the developmentally vulnerable period of childhood. Judges and juries will then take into account that the individual before them played no active role in bringing about the initial injury. However, the choices made later—for example, substance use and antisocial behavior—may lead to some degree of culpability.

Another source of misunderstanding among both mental health professionals and those outside the field is the notion that trauma and PTSD are synonymous. This is in large part due to psychiatric nomenclature where, even with the advent of *DSM-5*,[12] there are few diagnoses that require an etiology. Four diagnoses have potentially traumatizing experiences as a diagnostic criterion: reactive attachment disorder, acute stress disorder, PTSD, and adjustment disorders.[12,13] Given the criteria for these psychiatric disorders, it is difficult to diagnose with accuracy a child or adult with a history of numerous adverse and/or traumatic experiences presenting with multiple symptoms and difficulties but not meeting the threshold for PTSD. To capture the importance of their histories, these individuals are often (mis)diagnosed with PTSD (in addition to other disorders) to ensure that subsequent providers recognize the importance of their traumatic history as it relates to their presentation. Sometimes the forensic examiner will have to deconstruct the history of diagnostic labels to synthesize the case and meaningfully answer the consultation question.

While the misdiagnosis of PTSD begs the question of the overall utility of a descriptively derived nomenclature, it also leads to significant misunderstandings of people who are suffering from trauma-related issues, as well as their evaluation, treatment, and other therapeutic and supportive measures. This problem of misdiagnosis in a forensic report can lead to confusion in court.

While current estimates of PTSD range from about 10% to 20% in the general population,[14] for low socioeconomic groups and those seeking treatment for mental health issues, the estimates are closer to 40% to 50%.[15,16] PTSD, however, may not be the most common trauma-related diagnosis or problem for children and adolescents.[2–5] In adults, substance use disorders, depression, personality disorders, antisocial behavior, and other behavioral disturbances may be more common posttraumatic syndromes,[14] although they are not grouped with PTSD in *DSM-5*. While there are insufficient epidemiologic data about children and adolescents, there are known correlations between adolescent substance use and conduct disorder.[17,18] Children exposed to early maltreatment (e.g., children in the child welfare system) often have issues with attachment and behavioral problems, as well as cognitive and attentional difficulties.[19] Diagnoses such as complex PTSD[20] for adults and developmental trauma disorder[21,22] for children have been proposed to capture the complexity of these posttraumatic presentations but have not yet been included in the psychiatric nosology. This makes it essential that the expert witness convey a narrative connecting psychological trauma to subsequent behaviors, despite the limitations of the *DSM-5*. Nevertheless, the witness must be prepared to support any formal diagnosis with evidence.

It is now widely recognized that PTSD represents a traumatic injury to the brain with lasting impacts on behavioral function, but this diagnosis only captures a portion of the potential injury to brain function by the broader category of adverse experiences and chronic stress. The most insidious and widespread injuries to the brain are those caused by cumulative adverse experiences or unmediated stress. These too can result in trauma and behavioral disturbances.

CHILDHOOD MALTREATMENT AND CRIMINAL OFFENDING

We advise that expert witnesses in criminal cases be prepared to refer to literature on outcomes of traumatized children, especially when there is a challenge to the admissibility of testimony on the subject. Several studies highlight the disproportionate and enormous burden of exposure to ACEs among urban residents, youth in the juvenile justice system, and ultimately adults in the criminal justice system. More than 2,000 male and female first-grade students were recruited from a large city and interviewed later at a mean age of 21 to assess for the cumulative occurrence of traumatic events and the prevalence of PTSD.[23] Over 80% of the individuals reported one or more traumatic events. Of those who experienced a traumatic event, 60% were exposed to 4 or more. Nearly half of the sample experienced assaultive violence, and males were exposed to a greater risk of personal assaultive violence (58%), most often involving weapons. Females were at greater risk of rape. The overall conditional risk of PTSD was nearly 9%, with the risk of PTSD following assaultive violence the highest at 15%.

In another study of youth in the juvenile justice system from a large city, in a randomized sample of nearly 900 male and female youths, the investigators administered a standardized interview for trauma exposure and PTSD.[24] Greater than 90% of the sample reported at least 1 trauma, with 84% of those experiencing more than 1 and over half reporting 6 or more traumas; 11% were diagnosed with PTSD. The authors suggest that the standardized instrument used only focused on a single traumatic exposure and thus may have underestimated PTSD prevalence.

Beyond PTSD, there are other psychiatric sequelae of trauma exposure, and earlier studies have found that three quarters of female detainees and two thirds of male detainees have at least 1 psychiatric disorder,[25,26] with approximately half meeting criteria for 2 or more disorders.[27] These findings support the data suggesting that assessing for PTSD alone is insufficient to understand the impact of trauma and maltreatment among youth in the juvenile justice system. The range of trauma-related symptoms and behaviors unclassified as such in the *DSM-5* (and *DSM-IV*) forces the forensic psychiatrist to be versed in understanding and communicating these complexities to judges and juries.

A large retrospective, longitudinal study found that childhood maltreatment—including abuse and neglect—was a significant risk factor not only for juvenile delinquency but also for adult criminal behavior.[18] Over 900 individuals with substantiated childhood abuse and neglect were compared to 667 individuals without childhood abuse and were matched for age, sex, race, and family socioeconomic status. The investigators examined arrest records when the cohort averaged 26 years of age and again when the cohort averaged 32.5 years. At this later time point, greater than 99% of the subjects had passed through the peak offending years. The individuals who suffered childhood maltreatment were more likely to have been arrested as juveniles (27%) than those without a history of childhood abuse (17%). A greater proportion of the abused cohort were arrested as adults (42% v. 33%) and for violent crime (18% v. 14%). Those who had suffered abuse and neglect offended at nearly twice the rate, were arrested more frequently, and were younger at first arrest. In females, abuse and neglect increased the risk not only of criminal behavior, but also for committing violence. In males abuse and neglect did not increase the risk for violent offending. However, males who had suffered childhood maltreatment had a significantly greater number of arrests for violence than controls. Finally, childhood neglect was nearly as significant a risk factor for juvenile and adult criminal behavior as childhood physical abuse. As discussed below, these data have significant implications for recommendations for sentencing, decertification, and disposition of juvenile offenders.

CHILDHOOD MALTREATMENT AND ADULT OUTCOMES: THE ACE STUDY

The ACE Study is the largest of its kind to examine the health and social effects of ACEs. It is an ongoing collaboration between the Centers for Disease Control and Kaiser Permanente, surveying over 17,000 adults in a California HMO. To date the response rate has been over 70% for identifying 10 adverse childhood experiences (Box 4.1), with follow-up on health records for medical and behavioral outcomes.[7] More than half the respondents had at least 1 ACE, with a quarter of participants reporting 2 or more ACEs. The ACE score is simply additive, with no weighting of the individual relationship of cause and effect. The most significant finding was a graded relationship between higher ACE scores and increased prevalence of adult diseases and health-risk behaviors. Compared to those with no exposure, individuals with 4 or more categories of childhood maltreatment had a 4- to 12-fold increased risk for alcoholism, drug abuse, depression, and suicide attempts.

While you were growing up, during your first 18 years of life:

1. Did a parent or other adult in the household **often or very often ...**

   Swear at you, insult you, put you down, or humiliate you?

   or

   Act in a way that made you afraid that you might be physically hurt?

2. Did a parent or other adult in the household **often or very often ...**

   Push, grab, slap, or throw something at you?

   or

   Ever hit you so hard that you had marks or were injured?

3. Did an adult or person at least 5 years older than you **ever ...**

   Touch or fondle you or have you touch their body in a sexual way?

   or

   Attempt or actually have oral, anal, or vaginal intercourse with you?

4. Did you **often or very often** feel that ...

   No one in your family loved you or thought you were important or special?

   or

   Your family didn't look out for each other, feel close to each other, or support each other?

5. Did you **often or very often** feel that ...

   You didn't have enough to eat, had to wear dirty clothes, and had no one to protect you?

   or

   Your parents were too drunk or high to take care of you or take you to the doctor if you needed it?

6. Were your parents **ever** separated or divorced?

7. Was your mother or stepmother:

   Often or very often pushed, grabbed, slapped, or had something thrown at her?

   or

   Sometimes, often, or very often kicked, bitten, hit with a fist, or hit with something hard?

   or

Ever repeatedly hit at least a few minutes or threatened with a gun or knife?

8. Did you live with anyone who was a problem drinker or alcoholic or who used street drugs?

9. Was a household member depressed or mentally ill, or did a household member attempt suicide?

10. Did a household member go to prison?

Now add up your "Yes" answers: _____ **This is your ACE Score.**

(Retrieved from: http://www.acestudy.org/ace_score)

Increased ACE exposure also increased risk for adult diseases, including heart disease, cancer, lung disease, and liver disease. Since its initial publication this group has generated over 40 scientific articles across a broad range of health outcomes and high-risk behaviors. These additional data analyses have found associations between high ACE scores and premature death, numerous physical conditions, teen pregnancy, sexually transmitted diseases, adult revictimization, tobacco use, and substance use, as well as high burdens of mental illness. Moreover, other groups have studied ACE factors in correlation with health and behavioral outcomes. Follow-up studies from other groups have also looked to refine the list of ACEs used to screen individuals, with improved correlation with risk for mental health disorders.[28]

Significantly, this study has been conducted on a group of insured, largely middle-class individuals. One could envision additional adverse experiences suffered commonly by impoverished individuals, such as homelessness and shelter living, foster care and child protective service involvement, and navigating through violent neighborhoods.

There is one study exploring the relationship between ACEs and criminality.[29] The ACE questionnaire was administered to 151 individuals referred for outpatient treatment following convictions for nonsexual child abuse, domestic violence, stalking, and sexual offenses. Their results were compared to a normative sample of men drawn from the ACE Study database (Fig. 4.1). Nearly half of the offender group (48%) had an ACE score of 4+ compared to only 13% of men in the general ACE Study. All 10 ACEs were found in higher proportions in the offender group than the general population, with 8 achieving statistical significance. Conversely, fewer than 10% of the offenders reported no ACEs, whereas 38% of the control sample had an ACE score of zero. A limitation of this study is that the control group was not drawn from a matched cohort that was administered the ACE survey under the same conditions as the offenders. These data for criminal offenses add to

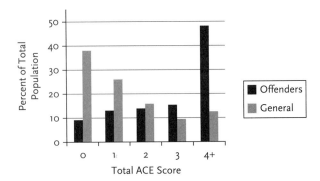

Fig. 4.1:
Results of the ACE questionnaire in offenders versus the general male population.
(Adapted from data in Reavis et al.[29])

the body of data demonstrating the increased risk of problem behaviors in adulthood for those with higher ACE scores. To the degree that mitigation testimony, for example, can assert that ACEs were experiences over which the defendant had no control, the dynamic may be persuasive. While especially salient in death-penalty situations, the information may also shape sentencing and other dispositional decisions before the court.

NEUROSCIENCE OF BRAIN CHANGES IN RESPONSE TO ACE

Childhood is a period of profound growth, when the developing brain responds to environmental influences to form lasting neuronal structures and connections that will regulate cognitive, emotional, and behavioral functioning. Multiple researchers have found that maltreatment affects a child's developing brain primarily through chronic overactivation of the stress response. This produces long-lasting alterations to brain structure and function, including changes in the corpus callosum and hippocampus as well as atypical electrical activity in multiple brain regions.[30] Studies are also beginning to examine how epigenetic mechanisms mediate the interplay between different environmental stressors and individual genomic differences that result in differences in long-term outcomes.[30] At this time, these research findings can be included as background for expert reports and testimony, although it would be premature to draw any conclusions about individuals.

Neuroanatomic Correlates

Childhood maltreatment activates the neurochemical and hormonal stress-response systems. The hypothalamic-pituitary-adrenal (HPA) axis is a central network of the stress-response systems, and its dysregulation is one of the key neurobiologic features of major depression, PTSD, and other psychiatric disturbances. Following HPA axis dysregulation, downstream effects are then seen on neurogenesis, synaptic pruning, and myelination. The major structural consequences include defects in the limbic system (temporal lobe, hippocampus, and amygdala), responsible for memory and emotional regulation, as well as the frontal cortex, involved in higher brain functions, such as personality, planning, judgment, social interaction, and behavioral control.

Neuroimaging studies of children with PTSD from maltreatment demonstrate a reduced volume of prefrontal white matter, right temporal lobe, and corpus callosum.[31] Decreases in hippocampal volume have been observed in individuals with PTSD from childhood physical and sexual abuse[32] as well as childhood maltreatment.[33] Drawing an interesting parallel between structure and function, reduced visual cortex gray matter has been measured in adults who witnessed domestic violence during childhood.[34] Lasting structural and functional impairments in neurobiologic circuits provide a mechanistic explanation for the increased risk of developing several psychiatric disorders, including substance abuse, depression, and PTSD.[35-37] We emphasize that although the research was done on children with PTSD, this diagnostic group is simply representative of the manner in which maltreatment and ACEs generally disrupt brain development and functioning.

Epigenetics: Gene–Environment Interactions

To adapt to environmental influences, neurons are extremely flexible in their connections to other neurons and can regulate their sensitivity to signal reception and transmission. This is mediated in large part through epigenetic mechanisms. Epigenetics is the manner by which gene function is controlled without making changes to the primary genome. Through a series of changes either to the proteins packaging the DNA, called histones, or to the nucleotides themselves through methylation of cytosine nucleotides at C-G dinucleotide sequences, a cell can regulate whether a gene is actively transcribed, affecting the total output of the gene product (ultimately a protein). Moreover, epigenetic changes can be long lasting, well beyond the initial environmental stimulus that initiated the change, and may therefore alter and regulate gene transcription for the life of the cell.

In anthropomorphic terms, epigenetics is how a cell "remembers" long term what happened to it and what "program" of genes it should be producing. While an individual's genes are responsible for which proteins they produce, the epigenetic structure around these genes is responsible for whether these genes are expressed at all and, if so, at what levels and when. This is most easily understood when considering that at the cellular level an individual's liver cells, skin cells, and neurons all share the exact same genes, but the proteins and ultimately the structure and function of each cell vary dramatically based on the epigenetic regulation of those genes to express a particular pattern of gene products in specific amounts. Ultimately, epigenetic regulation of gene transcription underpins brain development[38-40] and learning and memory.[41,42]

Epigenetic modifications have been shown to be molecular mechanisms that link early life experiences with neuronal development and ultimately adult functioning.[43] Several scientific studies have validated this model and demonstrated epigenetic changes in response to early developmental trauma and linked these to epigenetic changes as well as to alterations in brain development and adult brain function and behavior. Thus, the wound of psychological trauma is initiated and may be localized at the molecular level to epigenetic changes in the genome of cells in critical neuroanatomic structures and pathways. As the technology evolves there may come a time when information at this level can be brought to bear on the behavior of individuals, although not necessarily to excuse culpable behavior. At present there is no "smoking gun" to link psychological trauma to epigenetics and then to specific behaviors. Therefore, as a general principle, such dynamics are best reserved for mitigation of culpability, such as death-penalty trials.

Lessons from Animal Models

The pioneering work in epigenetic programming of neurons in early development by environmental influence and its lasting effect on adult behavior was first performed in studies with rats and extended by translational research to humans. Rat mothers demonstrate stable individual differences between nurturing mothers that provide optimal care for their pups and low-nurturing mothers that do not. Pups raised by nurturing mothers have good stress regulation, due in part to HPA axis and stress-hormone regulation. Accordingly, nurtured pups with good stress regulation have more glucocorticoid receptors in the hypothalamus and the promoter region of this gene has epigenetic changes allowing for increased gene expression, while low-nurtured pups have the inverse. Nurturing mothers raise pups that go on to be high-nurturing mothers, while the pups of low-nurturing mothers become low-nurturing mothers. While this pattern would appear to be genetically inherited, cross-fostering studies in which the offspring of low-nurturing mothers are raised by nurturing mothers and vice versa show instead that nurturing behavior is *not genetically* transmitted but *is imprinted* during early development of the pup.[44] Thus, the pups of low-nurturing mothers who were raised by nurturing foster mothers will develop into nurturing mothers and demonstrate the same epigenetic modifications at the glucocorticoid receptor gene that allowed for higher gene expression. Conversely, the pups of nurturing mothers raised by foster low-nurturing mothers lack the epigenetic enhancements and themselves become low-nurturing mothers.

The lasting effects of early maltreatment for epigenetic changes in pups have been established for other genes and other brain regions. Pups cross-fostered by stressed mother rats developed into adult rats with increased methylation of the gene for brain-derived neurotrophic factor (BDNF) and decreased expression of BDNF protein in the prefrontal cortex.[45] BDNF supports neuronal cell growth and survival[46] and plays a critical role in learning and memory.[47] These pups raised by low-nurturing, stressed mothers tend to have pups with altered epigenetic modifications and reduced BDNF expression.[45]

The amount of care a mother directs toward her female offspring also results in epigenetic changes to a specific type of estrogen receptor in the medial preoptic area, which is a brain region important for the expression of maternal care behaviors.[48] Early imprinting from maternal care also results in epigenetic changes to the estrogen receptor in the ventromedial nucleus of the hypothalamus, which is a part of the brain that controls sexual behaviors.[49] In cross-fostering studies, the female offspring of low-nurturing, stressed rat mothers are aggressive toward other females in competition for male suitors.[50] The female offspring of stressed rat mothers also have more sex, become pregnant more easily, and have more pups.[50] Females from low-care mothers also reach puberty earlier.[50]

Lessons from Human Studies

The impact of maternal behavior on gene methylation and expression has been extended to humans. McGowan and colleagues studied samples of brain tissue from men who had committed suicide and within this group compared those who had experienced childhood abuse and those who committed suicide but had not been abused.[51] A history of childhood abuse was determined though a structured assessment for psychological autopsies by chart reviews. Translating the findings with the glucocorticoid receptor in rats to humans, Van West and colleagues examined the homologous human glucocorticoid receptor gene, which is implicated in human studies with severe depression.[52] They found that the expression of the gene was significantly lower in abused men compared to nonabused men, and that this was reflected in differences in epigenetic modifications as well. In comparison, nonabused men who died by suicide and men who were neither abused nor committed suicide were not significantly different from each other in glucocorticoid gene expression or epigenetic modifications. This demonstrated in humans an epigenetic mechanism for linking the effects of early childhood trauma to gene expression and later adult mental and behavioral problems.

Building on the studies of single genes, whole-genome analyses of epigenetic modifications in maltreated children have been performed. Using institutionalization of children, a marker for early deprivation and maternal neglect, investigators compared children raised by their biologic parents of similar socioeconomic level by examining whole-genome methylation patterns from blood samples.[53] The institutionalized children were found to have increased levels of methylation relative to the comparison group, and the affected genes were primarily those involved in the immune response and cellular signaling, including several genes with known roles in brain development and function.[53] Another study looked at maltreated children who had been removed from their parents due to abuse or neglect, with 92% of them suffering multiple forms of maltreatment.[54] Compared to a demographically matched cohort of children without maltreatment, there were significant between-group differences in overall methylation patterns. Moreover, there were intergroup differences in methylation at disease biomarkers for several cancers.[54] Other investigators examined genome-wide DNA methylation changes in postmortem neuronal tissue from the hippocampus from men with a history of childhood abuse.[55] Severe childhood abuse was associated with several clusters of differentially methylated genes across multiple physiologic domains. However, genes involved in neuronal plasticity, which is the process by which neurons adapt and grow in relation to environmental stresses and changes, showed the greatest differences between the abused and nonabused men.[55]

An interesting study of genome-wide gene expression and epigenetic modifications examined individuals with PTSD and similar adult traumatic exposures and symptoms, but differing by types of childhood maltreatment experiences.[56] When the gene expression patterns were analyzed, they were almost completely nonoverlapping among the individuals with different childhood maltreatment exposures but similar PTSD symptoms. Comparing samples from individuals with PTSD who had suffered childhood maltreatment to DNA samples from individuals with PTSD who did not suffer childhood maltreatment, they found significantly different DNA methylation patterns at these gene loci. Thus, this study not only reinforced an epigenetic mechanism for the disturbances in PTSD but also suggested that even among those with a PTSD diagnosis, those with childhood maltreatment have a different set of genes involved, which may be related to developmental factors such as the greater plasticity of the brain in childhood. These studies in humans and animal models have demonstrated an epigenetic mechanism for transmitting the effects of early adverse experiences into deficits of later-life brain function and structure. We will now turn to the question of how this information could potentially be used in illuminating behavior in a legal setting.

CURRENT IMPACT ON FORENSIC ASSESSMENTS

Most treating and forensic psychiatrists routinely screen for the impact of early childhood emotional, physical, and sexual abuse and appreciate their impact on current functioning. The most important implication of the ACE Study for the forensic psychiatrist is that the 10 factors studied provide a broad range of potentially adverse childhood experiences. These factors, viewed as benign or irrelevant in isolation, when accumulated have a markedly negative impact on the developing young brain and body. The cumulative effect of even more seemingly benign factors, such as parental separation, lack of feeling special in the family, mental illness in a family member, or the incarceration of a family member, should be included in the formulation. The forensic examiner who does not at a minimum screen for the ACE factors or cumulative unmediated stress, in addition to other potentially traumatic experiences, has not performed a complete assessment of developmental history that may be especially salient for responding to legal questions of culpability and disposition.

Criminal Sentencing and Mitigation

The situation in which knowledge regarding child adversity and trauma may be most relevant is in the sentencing phase, especially death-penalty cases. Given that the death penalty is intended as punishment for those individuals who are the most morally culpable, an evaluation for psychological trauma and damages from early childhood maltreatment is most salient for mitigation. In a trio of cases addressing the constitutionality of penalties in juveniles, the U.S. Supreme Court considered scientific evidence concerning brain development in adolescents in arriving at their ruling that the death penalty is unconstitutional for juvenile offenders and in setting limits on sentencing juveniles to life without parole.[57-59] Similarly, the cumulative data from numerous epidemiologic studies, neuroanatomic studies, and studies of epigenetic molecular changes in brain physiology in response to early childhood maltreatment and abuse may be used by the forensic psychiatrist to educate the court concerning the impact of an individual's history of childhood maltreatment on subsequent mental functioning. Furthermore, by focusing on the full spectrum of accumulated adverse experiences and not more narrowly on single traumatic events or a PTSD diagnosis, the expert witness will be better able to recognize these relevant factors in a broader range of individuals who have committed criminal offenses. The accumulated knowledge can then be leveraged in the discussion of the individual in question.

Another opportunity for the forensic psychiatrist to educate the courts in the presentencing evaluation is to propose treatment recommendations that would both directly benefit the individual as well as potentially lower recidivism. A recognition of the pervasive negative influence of ACEs is most salient for engaging trauma-based therapies as the appropriate treatment modality for these complex cases of victims of childhood maltreatment that do not fit neatly into classic psychiatric syndromes.[60] This would be of particular importance to evaluations of juvenile offenders, where identification of the full spectrum of adverse experiences and their strong correlation with violence and criminal behavior can inform rehabilitation recommendations. Trauma-focused cognitive behavioral therapy (TF-CBT) is an effective evidence-based treatment for child victims of traumatic exposures and is not limited to those diagnosed with PTSD.[61-63] It has been proven effective in numerous populations, including children with behavioral problems[64] and incarcerated boys.[65] Moreover, in adults there is evidence for the effectiveness of numerous trauma-based therapies over standard therapies for individuals with trauma histories.[66-69] Whether the ultimate disposition is release into the community or incarceration, trauma-based treatments offer the opportunity to modify the negative influences of traumatic experiences on behavior and potentially reduce recidivism. This is especially important when the defendant's history is argued by the prosecution as evidence of an aggravating factor that is unlikely to be modified by available therapies.

Juvenile Court Applications

For juvenile offenders, a more complete assessment of the trauma history and knowledge of its impact on later adult criminal behavior can aid the forensic examiner in making recommendations to the court regarding the disposition of juvenile offenders, particularly in assessments for decertification proceedings, wherein the juvenile is arguing against trial in adult criminal court. Evidence of cumulative ACEs does raise the overall risk that the juvenile offender will reoffend as an adult. Furthermore, the evidence for the impact of chronic stress, trauma, and adverse experiences on normal childhood development is not conducive to tidy, simplistic assessments. On one hand, the traumatized youth may suffer delayed maturation of cognitive and emotional capacities, thus favoring decertification. On the other, ACEs may severely restrict such development, rendering it unlikely that further rehabilitative efforts in the juvenile system would succeed. The forensic psychiatrist performing decertification assessments, of course, must start with a solid foundation of expertise in childhood development. To that must be incorporated these data gathered here in order to comprehensively assess the impact of cumulative ACEs during different developmental stages for a particular individual. As with recommendations for adults, a familiarity with trauma-based therapies will enable the forensic psychiatrist to make recommendations to the court regarding a particular juvenile's potential for rehabilitation within the juvenile system. The expert's recommendations, then, will be based on clinical findings and guidance from research literature but will ultimately be framed in an individualized manner.

FUTURE IMPLICATIONS AND A FRAMEWORK FOR INCORPORATING NEW DATA

Studies continue to elucidate the many neuroanatomic and neurophysiologic sequelae of childhood trauma with greater precision in localizing the lesions at the molecular level, the structural level and the neurologic circuits involved. The next area of research will be extending these studies to examine the relationship between injuries from both devastating single traumatic events and multiple ACEs and establishing the relationship to the range of negative psychosocial and functional outcomes. Molecular studies have already traced these traumatic injuries to the level of epigenetic modifications of the genome, and further research will likely elucidate whether there is a final common pathway for multiple adverse experiences and traumas or whether different traumas and maltreatment have unique effects on the brain and behavior. Understanding differential epigenetic modifications may not only provide an explanation for individual differences in vulnerability and resiliency, but also offer promising therapeutic targets for preventing or reversing traumatic injuries.

A critical area for future research for forensic psychiatry would be to extend the analysis of the ACE Study to criminal behavior. The negative effects of multiple, cumulative childhood stressors on physical and mental health outcomes as well as harmful behaviors such drug addiction have been well established. At present, one can demonstrate a common pathway to delinquency and criminality using the ACE methodology: that high ACE scores greatly increase the risk of substance use, which is highly linked to future criminal behaviors. Direct examination using ACE criteria and similar structured assessments is likely to find a similar impact upon juvenile delinquency and adult criminal behavior. There is significant overlap among populations with substance use problems, behavioral disturbance, and criminal involvement. There is also the potential for additional large-scale studies further elucidating the link between childhood maltreatment and later delinquency and criminal behavior. This would lead not only to an understanding of the antecedents of behavioral problems, but also to the development of therapeutic interventions, including ones tailored to a juvenile or correctional setting. One potential intervention might be for a public defender's office to employ the ACE questionnaire as a screening tool, where defendants scoring 4 or higher were referred on for neuropsychiatric testing and forensic evaluation.

Ultimately we envision that future studies will allow the clinician and forensic examiner to describe a reasonable physiologic sequence from early childhood maltreatment to damage to individual molecular, epigenetic, neurotransmitter, and neuroanatomic circuits that result in specific behaviors demonstrated by certain individuals involved in criminal behaviors. For now, we can say that the science clearly supports a link between early childhood trauma and maltreatment and dysregulated development of cognitive, neuropsychiatric, and emotional pathways. These dysregulated pathways are more vulnerable to stressors, and these individuals are more likely to react with aberrant or even criminal behavior at lower thresholds. Thus, the current science clearly supports the presentation of early childhood maltreatment and trauma as relevant mitigating factors to be considered in the penalty phase of trials.

REFERENCES

1. Thornberry TP, Henry KL, Ireland TO, Smith CA. The causal impact of childhood-limited maltreatment and adolescent maltreatment on early adult adjustment. *J Adolesc Health*. 2010; 46(4): 359–365.
2. Fowler PJ, Tompsett CJ, Braciszewski JM, Jacques-Tiura AJ, Baltes BB. Community violence: a meta-analysis on the effect of exposure and mental health outcomes of children and adolescents. *Dev Psychopathol*. 2009; 21(1): 227–259.
3. Herrenkohl TI, Kosterman R, Mason WA, Hawkins JD. Youth violence trajectories and proximal characteristics of intimate partner violence. *Violence Vict*. 2007; 22(3): 259–274.
4. Putnam FW. Commentary on "Seven institutionalized children and their adaptation in late adulthood: The children of Duplessis." *Psychiatry*. 2006; 69(4): 333–335.
5. Scheeringa MS, Zeanah CH, Myers L, Putnam FW. New findings on alternative criteria for PTSD in preschool children. *J Am Acad Child Adolesc Psychiatry*. 2003; 42(5): 561–570.
6. Edwards VJ, Holden GW, Felitti VJ, Anda RF. Relationship between multiple forms of childhood maltreatment and adult mental health in community respondents: results from the Adverse Childhood Experiences Study. *Am J Psychiatry*. 2003; 160(8): 1453–1460.
7. Felitti VJ, Anda RF, Nordenberg D, et al. Relationship of childhood abuse and household dysfunction to many of the leading causes of death in adults. The Adverse Childhood Experiences (ACE) Study. *Am J Prev Med*. 1998; 14(4): 245–258.

8. Kandel ER. Psychotherapy and the single synapse. the impact of psychiatric thought on neurobiologic research. *N Engl J Med*. 1979; 301(19): 1028–1037.

9. Anda RF, Felitti VJ, Bremner JD, et al. The enduring effects of abuse and related adverse experiences in childhood. A convergence of evidence from neurobiology and epidemiology. *Eur Arch Psychiatry Clin Neurosci*. 2006; 256(3): 174–186.

10. Dong M, Anda RF, Felitti VJ, et al. The interrelatedness of multiple forms of childhood abuse, neglect, and household dysfunction. *Child Abuse Negl*. 2004; 28(7): 771–784.

11. Marans S, Adelman A. Experiencing violence in a developmental context. *Children in a Violent Society*. 1997: 202–222.

12. American Psychiatric Association. *DSM-5*. Washington, DC: American Psychiatric Association; 2013.

13. American Psychiatric Association. *Diagnostic and Statistical Manual of Mental Disorders: DSM-IV-TR®*. Washington, DC: American Psychiatric Publishing; 2000.

14. Breslau N. The epidemiology of trauma, PTSD, and other posttrauma disorders. *Trauma Violence Abuse*. 2009; 10(3): 198–210.

15. Horowitz K, McKay M, Marshall R. Community violence and urban families: experiences, effects, and directions for intervention. *Am J Orthopsychiatry*. 2005; 75(3): 356–368.

16. Schwartz AC, Bradley RL, Sexton M, Sherry A, Ressler KJ. Posttraumatic stress disorder among African Americans in an inner city mental health clinic. *Psychiatr Serv*. 2005; 56(2): 212–215.

17. White HR, Widom CS. Does childhood victimization increase the risk of early death? A 25-year prospective study. *Child Abuse Negl*. 2003; 27(7): 841–853.

18. Widom CS, Maxfield MG. *An Update on the "Cycle of Violence."* U.S. Department of Justice, Office of Justice Programs, National Institute of Justice; 2001.

19. Burke NJ, Hellman JL, Scott BG, Weems CF, Carrion VG. The impact of adverse childhood experiences on an urban pediatric population. *Child Abuse Negl*. 2011; 35(6): 408–413.

20. Roth S, Newman E, Pelcovitz D, van der Kolk B, Mandel FS. Complex PTSD in victims exposed to sexual and physical abuse: results from the DSM-IV field trial for posttraumatic stress disorder. *J Trauma Stress*. 1997; 10(4): 539–555.

21. Stolbach BC, Minshew R, Rompala V, Dominguez RZ, Gazibara T, Finke R. Complex trauma exposure and symptoms in urban traumatized children: a preliminary test of proposed criteria for developmental trauma disorder. *J Trauma Stress*. 2013; 26(4): 483–491.

22. Schmid M, Petermann F, Fegert JM. Developmental trauma disorder: pros and cons of including formal criteria in the psychiatric diagnostic systems. *BMC Psychiatry*. 2013; 13: 3-244X–13-3.

23. Breslau N, Wilcox HC, Storr CL, Lucia VC, Anthony JC. Trauma exposure and posttraumatic stress disorder: a study of youths in urban America. *J Urban Health*. 2004; 81(4): 530–544.

24. Abram KM, Teplin LA, Charles DR, Longworth SL, McClelland GM, Dulcan MK. Posttraumatic stress disorder and trauma in youth in juvenile detention. *Arch Gen Psychiatry*. 2004; 61(4): 403–410.

25. Teplin LA, Abram KM, McClelland GM, Dulcan MK, Mericle AA. Psychiatric disorders in youth in juvenile detention. *Arch Gen Psychiatry*. 2002; 59(12): 1133–1143.

26. Wasserman GA, McReynolds LS, Lucas CP, Fisher P, Santos L. The voice DISC-IV with incarcerated male youths: prevalence of disorder. *J Am Acad Child Adolesc Psychiatry*. 2002; 41(3): 314–321.

27. Abram KM, Teplin LA, McClelland GM, Dulcan MK. Comorbid psychiatric disorders in youth in juvenile detention. *Arch Gen Psychiatry*. 2003; 60(11): 1097–1108.

28. Finkelhor D, Shattuck A, Turner H, Hamby S. Improving the Adverse Childhood Experiences Study Scale. *JAMA Pediatr*. 2013; 167(1): 70–75.

29. Reavis JA, Looman J, Franco KA, Rojas B. Adverse childhood experiences and adult criminality: how long must we live before we possess our own lives? *Perm J*. 2013; 17(2): 44–48.

30. McCrory E, De Brito SA, Viding E. Research review: the neurobiology and genetics of maltreatment and adversity. *J Child Psychol Psychiatry*. 2010; 51(10): 1079–1095.

31. De Bellis MD, Keshavan MS, Shifflett H, et al. Brain structures in pediatric maltreatment-related posttraumatic stress disorder: a sociodemographically matched study. *Biol Psychiatry*. 2002; 52(11): 1066–1078.

32. Bremner JD, Randall P, Vermetten E, et al. Magnetic resonance imaging-based measurement of hippocampal volume in posttraumatic stress disorder related to childhood physical and sexual abuse—a preliminary report. *Biol Psychiatry*. 1997; 41(1): 23–32.

33. Teicher MH, Anderson CM, Polcari A. Childhood maltreatment is associated with reduced volume in the hippocampal subfields CA3, dentate gyrus, and subiculum. *Proc Natl Acad Sci USA*. 2012; 109(9): E563–E572.

34. Tomoda A, Polcari A, Anderson CM, Teicher MH. Reduced visual cortex gray matter volume and thickness in young adults who witnessed domestic violence during childhood. *PLoS One*. 2012; 7(12): e52528.

35. Teicher MH, Andersen SL, Polcari A, Anderson CM, Navalta CP. Developmental neurobiology of childhood stress and trauma. *Psychiatr Clin North Am*. 2002; 25(2): 397–426, vii–viii.

36. Beers SR, De Bellis MD. Neuropsychological function in children with maltreatment-related posttraumatic stress disorder. *Am J Psychiatry*. 2002; 159(3): 483–486.

37. Teicher MH, Andersen SL, Polcari A, Anderson CM, Navalta CP, Kim DM. The neurobiological consequences of early stress and childhood maltreatment. *Neurosci Biobehav Rev*. 2003; 27(1–2): 33–44.

38. Feng J, Fouse S, Fan G. Epigenetic regulation of neural gene expression and neuronal function. *Pediatr Res*. 2007; 61(5 Pt 2): 58R–63R.

39. Roth TL. Epigenetics of neurobiology and behavior during development and adulthood. *Dev Psychobiol*. 2012; 54(6): 590–597.

40. Maze I, Noh KM, Allis CD. Histone regulation in the CNS: basic principles of epigenetic plasticity. *Neuropsychopharmacology*. 2013; 38(1): 3–22.

41. Levenson JM, Sweatt JD. Epigenetic mechanisms in memory formation. *Nat Rev Neurosci*. 2005; 6(2): 108–118.

42. Zovkic IB, Guzman-Karlsson MC, Sweatt JD. Epigenetic regulation of memory formation and maintenance. *Learn Mem*. 2013; 20(2): 61–74.

43. Murgatroyd C, Spengler D. Epigenetics of early child development. *Front Psychiatry*. 2011; 2: 16.

44. Weaver IC, Cervoni N, Champagne FA, et al. Epigenetic programming by maternal behavior. *Nat Neurosci*. 2004; 7(8): 847–854.

45. Roth TL, Lubin FD, Funk AJ, Sweatt JD. Lasting epigenetic influence of early-life adversity on the BDNF gene. *Biol Psychiatry*. 2009; 65(9): 760–769.
46. Huang EJ, Reichardt LF. Neurotrophins: roles in neuronal development and function. *Annu Rev Neurosci*. 2001; 24: 677–736.
47. Bekinschtein P, Cammarota M, Katche C, et al. BDNF is essential to promote persistence of long-term memory storage. *Proc Natl Acad Sci USA*. 2008; 105(7): 2711–2716.
48. Champagne FA, Weaver IC, Diorio J, Sharma S, Meaney MJ. Natural variations in maternal care are associated with estrogen receptor alpha expression and estrogen sensitivity in the medial preoptic area. *Endocrinology*. 2003; 144(11): 4720–4724.
49. Cameron NM, Soehngen E, Meaney MJ. Variation in maternal care influences ventromedial hypothalamus activation in the rat. *J Neuroendocrinol*. 2011; 23(5): 393–400.
50. Cameron N, Del Corpo A, Diorio J, McAllister K, Sharma S, Meaney MJ. Maternal programming of sexual behavior and hypothalamic-pituitary-gonadal function in the female rat. *PLoS One*. 2008; 3(5): e2210.
51. McGowan PO, Sasaki A, D'Alessio AC, et al. Epigenetic regulation of the glucocorticoid receptor in human brain associates with childhood abuse. *Nat Neurosci*. 2009; 12(3): 342–348.
52. van West D, Van Den Eede F, Del-Favero J, et al. Glucocorticoid receptor gene-based SNP analysis in patients with recurrent major depression. *Neuropsychopharmacology*. 2006; 31(3): 620–627.
53. Naumova OY, Lee M, Koposov R, Szyf M, Dozier M, Grigorenko EL. Differential patterns of whole-genome DNA methylation in institutionalized children and children raised by their biological parents. *Dev Psychopathol*. 2012; 24(1): 143–155.
54. Yang BZ, Zhang H, Ge W, et al. Child abuse and epigenetic mechanisms of disease risk. *Am J Prev Med*. 2013; 44(2): 101–107.
55. Labonté B, Suderman M, Maussion G, et al. Genome-wide epigenetic regulation by early-life trauma. *Arch Gen Psychiatry*. 2012; 69(7): 722–731.
56. Mehta D, Klengel T, Conneely KN, et al. Childhood maltreatment is associated with distinct genomic and epigenetic profiles in posttraumatic stress disorder. *Proc Natl Acad Sci USA*. 2013; 110(20): 8302–8307.
57. *Roper* v. *Simmons*. 543 U.S. 551, 125 S. Ct. 1183, 161 L. Ed. 2d 1 (2005).
58. *Graham* v. *Florida*, 130 S. Ct. 2011, 560 U.S. 48, 176 L. Ed. 2d 825 (2010).
59. *Miller* v. *Alabama*, 132 S. Ct. 2455, 567 U.S., 183 L. Ed. 2d 407 (2012).
60. Berkowitz SJ. Childhood trauma and adverse experience and forensic child psychiatry: The Penn Center for Youth and Family Trauma Response and Recovery. *J Psychiatry Law*. 2012; 40(1): 5–22.
61. Silverman WK, Ortiz CD, Viswesvaran C, et al. Evidence-based psychosocial treatments for children and adolescents exposed to traumatic events. *J Clin Child Adolesc Psychol*. 2008; 37(1): 156–183.
62. Cohen JA, Mannarino AP. Psychotherapeutic options for traumatized children. *Curr Opin Pediatr*. 2010; 22(5): 605–609.
63. Smith P, Perrin S, Dalgleish T, Meiser-Stedman R, Clark DM, Yule W. Treatment of posttraumatic stress disorder in children and adolescents. *Curr Opin Psychiatry*. 2013; 26(1): 66–72.
64. Cohen JA, Berliner L, Mannarino A. Trauma-focused CBT for children with co-occurring trauma and behavior problems. *Child Abuse Negl*. 2010; 34(4): 215–224.

65. Leenarts LE, Diehle J, Doreleijers TA, Jansma EP, Lindauer RJ. Evidence-based treatments for children with trauma-related psychopathology as a result of childhood maltreatment: a systematic review. *Eur Child Adolesc Psychiatry.* 2013; 22(5): 269–283.
66. Bisson J, Andrew M. Psychological treatment of post-traumatic stress disorder (PTSD). *Cochrane Database Syst Rev.* 2007; (3)(3): CD003388.
67. Bisson JI, Ehlers A, Matthews R, Pilling S, Richards D, Turner S. Psychological treatments for chronic post-traumatic stress disorder: systematic review and meta-analysis. *Br J Psychiatry.* 2007; 190: 97–104.
68. Ponniah K, Hollon SD. Empirically supported psychological treatments for adult acute stress disorder and posttraumatic stress disorder: a review. *Depress Anxiety.* 2009; 26(12): 1086–1109.
69. Ehlers A, Bisson J, Clark DM, et al. Do all psychological treatments really work the same in posttraumatic stress disorder? *Clin Psychol Rev.* 2010; 30(2): 269–276.

CHAPTER 5

Autism Spectrum Disorder and Criminal Justice

KENNETH J. WEISS AND ALEXANDER R. N. WESTPHAL*

The term *autism* was first used in a clinical context by Eugen Bleuler to describe the withdrawal from the social world that accompanied schizophrenia.[1] Many years later, Leo Kanner and Hans Asperger used it almost simultaneously to describe children referred to them because of profound social disabilities and rigid and repetitive patterns of behavior.[2,3] Since the 1980s, the various diagnostic systems used by mental health professionals have included a number of autism-related diagnoses, a reflection of the dimensional heterogeneity of presentations. These have included Asperger disorder, pervasive developmental disorder, autistic disorder, and childhood disintegrative disorder. However, the fifth edition of the *Diagnostic and Statistical Manual of Mental Disorders* of the American Psychiatric Association (*DSM-5*),[4] the most widely used diagnostic system, has eliminated all diagnoses but a single "autism spectrum disorder," with the rationale that the previous criteria used to distinguish them were insufficiently categorical, "equivalent to trying to 'cleave meatloaf at the joints'."[5]

Autism spectrum disorder (ASD), as defined in the *DSM-5*, is characterized by deficits in social communication and interaction, together with restricted or repetitive patterns of behavior. At its heart, it is a disorder of social relatedness. Descriptions associating ASD with unlawful behavior date back to Hans Asperger's early description of autism ("autistic psychopathy"). Among Asperger's subjects were four children referred to his clinic because of

---

* Portions of this chapter were previously published as: Weiss KJ. Autism spectrum disorder and criminal justice: Square peg in a round hole? *Am J Forensic Psychiatry.* 2011; 32(3): 3–19. Used with permission from the American College of Forensic Psychiatry, Carlsbad, CA.

problematic conduct in school. Of one of the subjects Asperger wrote, "[He] did not know the meaning of respect and was utterly indifferent to the authority of adults" (p. 86). He concluded, "The nature of these children is revealed most clearly in their behavior towards other people. Indeed, their behavior in the social group is the clearest sign of their disorder" (p. 121).[3]

ASD AND CRIMINAL JUSTICE

Persons with ASD encounter criminal justice for a variety of reasons: as a victim or a witness, or when accused of a criminal act. Given that criminal justice systems exist to govern social behaviors, it is not surprising that a disability in social cognition and judgment could impair the ability to conform one's behaviors to the law. Moreover, some of the core features of ASD, such as impaired communication and social skills, circumscribed interests, and deficits in abstract thought, may also undermine social adaptation.

The literature on the overlap between autism and criminal behavior is, however, limited and largely anecdotal. There is some primary research on the topic, but in a recent review Mouridsen concluded that the "results published so far [provide] no basis for addressing whether an association exists between ASD and offending" (p. 81). [6] Meanwhile, sensationalistic news reporting—often cloaked as science—has magnified single cases, obscuring what is actually known. Thus the expert witness may have two jobs: to educate courts about ASD and to dispel myths.

Deviance with a Difference

When people with ASD do offend, the reasons may be different from those of a typical offender. The term *counterfeit deviance* describes inappropriate sexual behavior rooted in factors such as sexual and social naïveté rather than in a paraphilia or sexual aggression.[7] Attorney Mark Mahoney applied the concept to criminal actions in people with autism, advising, "When an individual with [ASD] is accused of deviance or a sexual offense, a careful assessment must be conducted to determine if a Paraphilia is indeed present, which is not impossible, or if the differential diagnosis of counterfeit deviance applies" (p. 27). [8] We believe, as Mahoney does, that it is incumbent on defense attorneys and their expert witnesses to be able to convey alternate narratives to a case, when they are applicable. There is an art to forensic evaluations of defendants with ASD because of the need to explain the behaviors that led to the legal trouble in the context of the social disability. When assisting the prosecution, the expert witness can assess the strength of the defense claim, helping to guide the court as to whether the disorder forms the basis of a defense or mitigation.

The concept of *counterfeit deviance* is generalizable beyond sexual behavior. Take, for example, the case of Darius McCollum, discussed in Wendy Murphy's book, *Orphan Diseases*,[9] who has spent a large amount of his adult life incarcerated for stealing (and in most cases returning) transit vehicles. McCollum's behavior was clearly rooted in his restricted and highly focused interest in transit systems and enabled by the absence of checks that intact social insight would provide. However, the fact that he had been incarcerated repeatedly indicated that the legal system believed he should be punished for his actions in the same way as someone who committed the acts for a criminal purpose.

Understanding Differences

Another example of an ASD-related focused interest that led to legal trouble is described in *Raising Cubby: A Father and Son's Adventures with Asperger's, Trains, Tractors, and High Explosives*.[10] In the book, John Elder Robison discusses his son Cubby's specialized interest in explosive chemicals and his arrest after he posted footage of the explosions on the Internet. The investigation and court proceedings were dramatic, highlighting many of the issues discussed in this chapter, and are the subject of thorough descriptions by Robison. Ultimately Cubby was absolved of the charges.

One of the most important ways to protect people with ASD from situations like Robison's and McCollum's is to reduce behaviors that might lead them to legal trouble. To this end, problem behaviors should be addressed as they arise, and efforts should be made to direct behaviors to less maladaptive ends. The publishing house Diverse City Press provides excellent resources focused on sexual behaviors in particular.[11] In addition, preparation to prevent situations from escalating is essential. Dennis Debbaudt, the father of a person with ASD and a retired member of law enforcement, has developed trainings for law enforcement officials to recognize and interact with people who have ASD. He has also developed trainings for parents and care providers to reduce the likelihood that interactions with law enforcement escalate; they are available online.[12]

In summary, law is a mechanism by which social behaviors are codified and held to an acceptable standard. ASD undermines social insight and consequently may be associated with legal trouble. Some of these problematic behaviors may reflect drives and motivations that are quite different from the antisocial drives that the surface behaviors suggest, and their expression may reflect a lack of insight into how the behavior may appear to others. When someone with autism is in trouble, healthcare professionals can often play an important role in the legal process by explaining to the legal system that some behaviors that might appear to be driven by personal gain or other antisocial ends might actually reflect the disability in social insight that defines autism. In the sections to follow, we will discuss the uneasy intersection between ASD and the criminal justice system, giving examples of news stories and case law that illustrate some of the challenges that may confront those involved in the evaluations of defendants with ASD.

ASD AND CRIME: CONNECTING THE DOTS

When the psychiatric expert witness is called by the defense to explain the behavior of a defendant with ASD, the principal task is to link known autistic behaviors with plausible adaptive responses. From a diagnostic point of view, the defining feature of ASD is an abnormality of social behavior.[4] Underlying this is a disability in social cognition, especially in the area of empathy or Theory of Mind (ToM, "mentalizing"). In a cultural milieu where citizens are asked to report "suspicious behavior," it is not difficult to see how oddly behaving children and adults can become the focus of concern.

Deficits in Social Cognition

A recent cinematic example comes from the movie *Adam*, which portrays the adaptations of a young man with ASD in social, vocational, and sexual domains.[13] In one scene, Adam gets fired from his job after a meltdown. A bit disoriented and carrying a carton with his office artifacts, he finds himself alongside a schoolyard, staring at the children during recess. The police pull up in a car, and when they ask him what he is doing, he guilelessly replies, "Watching the children." Someone had called the police thinking Adam might be a pervert, but he is saved when his neighbor, a teacher at the school, recognizes him and tells the police she knows him.

Not all situations resolve as smoothly. Individuals with ASD may become easily flustered in confrontations with law enforcement. Under some circumstances, difficulties with emotion regulation can cause them to appear highly threatening. In South Carolina in 2009, a 15-year-old boy with Asperger disorder was fatally shot after pulling a knife and attacking a school resource officer. On the basis of the case, the NAACP called for training of law enforcement officials about ASD.[14] Similar situations have prompted calls for mandatory training of police in recognizing and handling individuals with ASD.[15]

Even when law enforcement does recognize the presence of an ASD, problems can arise. In *Ohio v. Eal*,[16] the court considered and rejected the defendant's claim that the arresting officers' style of questioning was inherently coercive because the officers were aware of the defendant's Asperger disorder, carried firearms, and isolated the defendant from his parents during the interview. Furthermore, in support of his claim that the interview was coercive, Eal argued that the nature of his Asperger disorder caused his developmental age to be lower than his chronological age: "Although defendant was 19 years old at the time of the interview, defendant asserts that, as a result of his Asperger's syndrome, he was interacting and understanding the world like a 14, 15, 16-year-old." The court wrote that "even assuming the officers were aware of defendant's Asperger's Disorder at the time of the interview, mere knowledge of a defendant's mental condition does not prove that the law enforcement officials resorted to psychological pressure or tactics to coerce incriminating statements."[16] Although Eal was unsuccessful in his line of defense, the case established a precedent for considering that defendants with ASD may have particular vulnerabilities during interrogations.

ASD Phenotype: Looking Guilty

One of the most common features of ASD is the avoidance of eye contact. In the beginning of his memoir on living with Asperger disorder, Robison (p. 2)[17] recalled how such behavior leads to misattributions of untrustworthiness early in life: "Everyone thought they understood my behavior. They thought it was simple: I was just no good. 'Nobody trusts a man who won't look them in the eye'. 'You look like a criminal'. 'You're up to something. I know it!' Most of the time, I wasn't. I didn't know why they were getting agitated. I didn't even understand what looking someone in the eye meant." On the principle that nonverbal behavior plays a big role in social judgments, one can easily see how the difficulties people with ASD have with social interactions can be misattributed to nefarious motives.

Inappropriate reactions to ordinary social situations may result in criminal penalties for persons with ASD. Allen and colleagues[18] looked at a sample (N = 16) of such individuals in the justice system, asking about precipitating factors and offending behaviors. Among the prominent clinical features of the offenders were lack of concern for outcome, social naïveté, and lack of awareness of outcome. Prominent precipitating factors to violence were social or sexual rejection and bullying. In a series of case examples, Schwartz-Watts[19] illustrated that individuals with tactile sensitivity, for example, may strike out violently when touched about the head or face. In one of the cases, the defendant with ASD had difficulty recognizing faces and facial cues, but the judge would not permit testimony on this point. Sentences for ASD defendants may also be harsher because they appear to lack remorse. Explaining an apparent lack of remorse can be an important role for an expert witness. For example, a Massachusetts teen with Asperger disorder was sentenced to life in prison for fatally stabbing another boy. Convicted after a failed insanity plea,[20] his argument for sentence reduction was also rejected.[21] Despite the defense bringing to the court's attention the unique qualities of ASD, the court sentenced the crime, not the person.

British criminal justice acknowledges individual differences and the possibility of early identification of vulnerable individuals. This is especially evident in a recent publication by the Prison Reform Trust, supported by the Diana, Princess of Wales Memorial Fund.[22] Compared with the one-size-fits-all model of retribution illustrated in the Massachusetts case, the British programs emphasize education of care providers and the establishment of alternate "offender pathways" for youths with learning disabilities or low IQ, communication difficulties, mental illness, attention-deficit disorder, and ASD.

In a parallel phenomenon, there was great public support for a Glasgow-born Londoner with Asperger disorder, Gary McKinnon, who hacked into the Pentagon's computers in search of evidence of UFOs. He was charged criminally in the United States, and his fight against extradition was in the newspapers and other media in the United Kingdom.[23,24] A "Free Gary" movement (freegary.org.uk) that attracted celebrities and a vigorous discussion in Parliament formed.[25,26] Ultimately the charges against McKinnon were dropped.

There are differences in the way *mens rea* is adjudicated in Britain and Australia. Relevant cases have been reviewed by Wauhop.[27] These adjudications take a broad approach to the inclusion of ASD evidence—for example, reduction in culpability, reduction in sentence, evidence of cognitive impairment, reduction in objective criminality, and reading social cues.[27] The recurrent themes (including American cases), according to Wauhop, include failure of proof defense, mistake in fact defense, and mitigation of offense level; the results are mixed.

ASD IN THE COURTS

Although it is not feasible to determine the frequency of using ASD as a diagnosis supporting a psychiatric defense to criminal charges, a Lexis Legal Research search for federal and state opinions yielded relatively few results. The following examples illustrate the various approaches used to educate courts about ASD and criminal responsibility. The cases emphasize the difficulties in reconciling clinical information with applicable standards.

The U.S. Court of Appeals for the Ninth Circuit dealt with an interesting set of facts in relation to social cognition, namely whether Asperger disorder would interfere with a defendant's ability to infer information that a crime would take place. In *U.S. v. Cottrell*[28] the defendant-appellant, a man with ASD, had been convicted of several counts each of conspiracy to commit arson and vandalism. Cottrell was barred by the trial court from presenting evidence of Asperger disorder. The Ninth Circuit appeals court agreed it was not relevant to an objective standard in relation to conspiracy: "Blindness may be taken into account in determining criminal responsibility, for example, because it limits the facts available to the defendant, but a condition like Asperger's, which affects only the defendant's ability to draw inferences from facts that he perceives, does not qualify" (p. 216).[28] Thus, it would not have been relevant to culpability whether Cottrell had a subjective belief that no further crimes would be committed. However, with respect to arson itself, the court ruled that, since it is a specific-intent crime, evidence of Asperger disorder was relevant; they vacated the arson convictions.

In a military case involving a conviction for giving intelligence to the enemy and related offenses, there were differing opinions as to the implications of Asperger disorder for cognitive functioning.[29] The defendant, Specialist Anderson, had posted comments on a website called "Brave Muslims" among other activities. At trial, he used the services of a clinical psychologist and an Army psychiatrist, while the government had a forensic psychiatrist. The appeal itself concerned a question of imbalance between the experts; the court ruled there was not. The Army psychiatrist, not the expert in psychology, diagnosed the soldier with Asperger and bipolar disorders, "which inhibited Appellant's ability to interact with others but did not affect his knowledge of the difference between right and wrong" (p. 382).[29] The government's forensic psychiatrist agreed that Asperger disorder affected social behavior but not cognitive functioning. It seems unlikely that the concept of "social cognition" entered into the analysis.

Explaining ASD: An Excuse?

A first-degree murder conviction was overturned in Missouri[30] after it was ruled that the trial court erred in excluding evidence of Asperger disorder. The defendant-appellant, Boyd, intended to use evidence of his condition to explain his unusually focused interest in violent books, his gullibility, and his susceptibility to being framed. His expert would have opined that Asperger disorder affects social cognition. In addition to claiming innocence, he wished to assert that his condition precluded the degree of physical coordination required for the murder and the ability to track through woods. The appellate court considered whether Boyd's evidence needed to be within the scope of mental disease defined under the diminished capacity statute, and decided it did not. Because the introduction of his evidence could have resulted in a different outcome, Boyd was granted a new trial.

A Texas man with Asperger disorder used an attack on *mens rea* in a case involving taking sexual photographs of teenage girls and other allegations.[31]

He appealed after being convicted of indecency and sentenced to 15 years in prison. Under Texas law there is no diminished capacity defense, only a failure of proof, including evidence to negate *mens rea*. At trial, the defendant, Pearce, proffered psychological testimony that he had Asperger disorder and a corresponding mental age of 13 to 16, thus rendering him a "peer" to the victims. The psychologist, however, did not draw a connection between this clinical finding and the question of criminal responsibility. Nevertheless, Pearce argued in the appeal that the jury should have been instructed on lesser-included offenses based on negation of *mens rea*. The appellate court rejected the appeal.

A Pennsylvania man attempted to use evidence of autism as the basis for an insanity defense to attempted homicide.[32] Instead, he was convicted under the guilty-but-mentally-ill statute. Whereas both sides agreed on the diagnosis, the forensic psychiatrist for the prosecution opined that the defendant, Daniel, only met the definition of "mentally ill," whereas the defense witness opined that autism prevented Daniel from knowing the wrongfulness of his conduct. Because the defendant argued an insanity defense, the jury also received instruction on guilty but mentally ill. The appeal was based on burden of proof and jury instruction. Accordingly, the opinion said little about the details of the defense testimony on autism and criminal responsibility.

Similarly, a case in Florida explored whether the presence of Asperger disorder was enough to evoke the constitutional bar on executing the intellectually disabled. Defendant Schoenwetter was sentenced to death after he was found guilty of killing two people and seriously injuring another in a home invasion. Among various proceedings, the court denied his petition for a writ of habeas corpus, which included the claim that evolving standards of decency as outlined in *Atkins v. Virginia* were relevant to him because he suffered from Asperger syndrome, attention-deficit/hyperactivity disorder, and frontal lobe damage. The court found that although the conditions might be mitigating, and noted that they were considered as such by the trial court, "mere mental illness does not serve as a bar to execution under *Atkins*."[33]

Admissibility and Rule 402

A criminal defendant with ASD, depending on jurisdiction, may not have an excuse based on a M'Naghten-type standard or a failure of proof via diminished capacity. However, the question has arisen whether it would be permitted to proffer expert testimony on clinical characteristics of a defendant and persons with ASD generally. While not used in the service of an affirmative defense, testimony would focus on providing the judge or jury with an alternate explanation of the defendant's behavior. This would give the fact finder an opportunity to decide whether, based on the subjective factors of the defendant at the time in question, the prosecution met its burden of proof beyond a reasonable doubt. Such a case was decided by the Supreme Court of New Jersey in 2008.[34]

The defendant, Burr, a children's music teacher with ASD, was accused of fondling a 7-year-old student over her clothing. The charges implied that he had "groomed" the child for these contacts and that he subjected her to humiliation. He claimed that he received no sexual gratification from the encounters and that the charges were not factual. Burr tried to bolster his defense by using a psychiatrist's testimony that Asperger disorder prevented him from having the nefarious motives attributed by the victims. The trial court did not permit it and Burr was convicted and sent to prison.

It is clear that the trial judge only considered the expert testimony in light of an attack on *mens rea*: "But I am satisfied there is no basis to have Doctor Kleinmann testify…as to the condition of Asperger's Syndrome. I don't know the relevance of his condition insofar as it relates to this case…[T]here is no…contention that [defendant] cannot formulate the mental attitude of purposefulness or knowledge sufficient to commit the crimes in question" (p. 551).[35] Burr appealed and the appellate court found that the trial court had erred in barring expert testimony, reversing the conviction and ordering a new trial.[35] That court stated, "Because the diminished capacity statute addresses only a narrow issue that is not applicable to these facts, evaluating the admissibility of defendant's Asperger's Disorder should have been guided by our more general rules of evidence" (p. 557).[35] The court concluded: "Clearly then, [Dr.] Kleinmann's testimony would have given jurors a better understanding of defendant's behavior, which could have effectively negated the inference that defendant had the improper motive of seeking sexual gratification by having children sit on his lap. The trial would have been a more fair and complete adversarial process if, in evaluating the evidence and the inferences urged by the State, jurors were aware that defendant's mental disability prevents him from viewing the world as others do in terms of acceptable social interactions" (p. 561).[35]

The prosecution appealed and, in 2008, the Supreme Court of New Jersey agreed to hear arguments. They upheld the appellate ruling granting Burr a new trial, saying that a defendant must be permitted to present any evidence relevant to explaining behavior, independent of whether it amounted to a formal psychiatric defense of diminished capacity. The basis of the ruling on expert testimony was New Jersey Rule of Evidence 402 (Relevant Evidence Generally Admissible), based on Federal Rule 402. The New Jersey high court's ruling distinguished the use of such evidence from the use of scientific evidence of mental disease to negate a specific element of an offense (diminished capacity), although in both cases the strategy is failure of proof. The practical difference is that, in diminished capacity, the defense essentially admits that the defendant committed the act, whereas in the *Burr* scenario the evidence only suggests how the characteristics of the defendant reduced the feasibility of the crime occurring.

When Burr was retried in 2010, the jury was hung on the sexual assault charge but convicted him on endangering the children. The State chose not to prosecute further. Nevertheless, the New Jersey precedent opens the door to clinical and other evidence of the characteristics of ASD that might be admissible in a variety of scenarios.

Informing Jurisprudence: More Examples

Several other cases have also discussed some of the issues highlighted by Burr. In *California v. Larsen*,[36] heard in the California court of appeal in 2012, the defendant was successful in arguing that the trial court infringed on his constitutional right to present a defense based on a purported mental impairment caused by Asperger syndrome, by refusing to give a specific mental disorder instruction to the jury. Larsen had been charged with soliciting the murder of a witness against him in an act for which he was incarcerated. The court's finding supported the conceptualization of Asperger disorder as a mental diagnosis that was relevant to the formation of specific intent and that had the potential to alter perceptions and mental processes in a way that undermined the ability to form intent. Although the appeals court concluded that the trial court's failure to deliver an instruction directing the jury's attention to the expert testimony of Asperger syndrome was an error, they also concluded that doing so would not have substantially altered the outcome of this particular trial (a reflection of the fact that they concluded that evidence of the defendant's guilt not only was compelling, but also did not alter his perceptions or mental processes in a way that was relevant) and so did not reverse the conspiracy or solicitation convictions.[36]

On the other hand, in *Minnesota v. Anderson*,[37] an appeal heard by the Supreme Court of Minnesota in 2010, it was found that the presence of Asperger disorder does not prevent a person from premeditating or forming intent. The defendant had been charged with killing a woman he had lured to his place with a fictional babysitting job. He contended that that his brain function was abnormal, and "by excluding the expert psychiatric testimony, the jurors inferred intent and premeditation based on an irrebuttable presumption that his brain was normal." He argued that he had a right to call witnesses to establish that his brain did not function normally, and furthermore that it was a denial of due process to exclude evidence of his mental disability. However, the court found that Anderson had withdrawn his mental illness defense by forgoing a bifurcated trial.[37]

Citing *Minnesota v. Bouwman*,[38] the court wrote, "[t]he law recognizes no degree of sanity. Applying socially and morally acceptable standards a line has been drawn—on one side are the legally sane, on the other side are the legally insane." Thus the court rejected Anderson's attempt to introduce expert testimony to link Asperger disorder to intent and premeditation, and furthermore established that it would have to qualify as "legal insanity" to be relevant.

EDUCATING COURTS ABOUT ASD

There is no legal principle that would shield a person with ASD from criminal prosecution, and none is endorsed here. The news accounts of prosecutions of ASD offenders suggest that, in America, the time is not ripe for inclusion of ASD in insanity defense considerations. Nevertheless, an attempt by the defense to educate the judge or jury about the characteristics of these individuals can aim at establishing reasonable doubt as to criminal intent and culpability. Using current research on ASD, the following are suggestions for types of scientific evidence that could underscore the nature of differences observed, without suggesting that persons with ASD are intrinsically incapable of criminal intent. These research studies may be used for inferences about specific defendants, but the fact that they are not definitive will aid expert witnesses on the prosecution side.

ToM and the Appearance of Evil

The behavioral phenotype of ASD has been characterized as an essential triad: deficits in reciprocal social behavior; verbal and nonverbal communication deficits; and stereotyped, repetitive, and highly focused activities. According to Haskins and Silva,[39] criminal behavior typically stems from two broad domains within these parameters: deficits in ToM (mentalization) and repetitive narrow interests. These traits are not conducive to earning the sympathy of lawyers, judges, jurors, or probation officers. In *McKinnon*, for example, when asked about his computer hacking, the defendant dismissed the American legal system and launched into a discussion of his narrowly focused interest—finding evidence of UFOs in government files. If one did not appreciate the nature of his extreme focus, it would appear that he was highly narcissistic and unwilling to accept the wrongfulness of his behavior. In *Burr*, although the defendant denied he had done anything wrong, the clinical evidence presented left the impression that it was unimaginable that one of his students would see his behavior as inappropriate—that is, he lacked the mentalizing ability to put himself in the child's place and acknowledge how she might have felt.

It would be important, when presenting testimony about the ASD phenotype, to emphasize the difference between cold, unfeeling behavior, on the one hand, and the type of deficit that reflects "mindblindness"[40] and interests that tend to exclude others' feelings. This is a difficult assignment, because the attitudes of judges and jurors may not permit the flexibility to operationalize ASD deficits in a way that distinguishes callousness rooted in psychopathy from a disability in social insight. Indeed, one can envision cross-examination based on the idea that ASD and psychopathy are kindred phenomena, since both entail empathy deficits. The defense expert witness would have to guard against taking this one trait out of context, whereas the prosecution witness might conflate the two types of psychopathology. Haskins and Silva emphasize this point in regard to phenotypic lack of remorse.[39] They acknowledge the possibility of ASD and psychopathy coexisting, as well as the opportunity to educate the court on ASD being "a neuropsychiatric developmental disorder with a high degree of heritability." In addition, they conclude that ToM may illuminate the analysis of intent, which is relevant to culpability.

Can Science Help?

There is growing literature on ASD in its many dimensions, even in the face of diagnostic ambiguity.[41] This, by itself, does not render the information admissible or relevant to the legal questions posed within criminal justice. As Silva[42] has pointed out, neuroscience has much to offer jurisprudence, although scientists must be careful not to confuse physiology with morality. That is, all behavior has dynamics and various levels of causation, but causes per se do little to inform the jurisprudence of responsibility. Taking our cue from a decision such as Burr, it is reasonable to ask what sorts of science might help juries and judges to consider degrees of blameworthiness, if not culpability, among persons with ASD. The following are a few examples drawn from the huge literature on developmental neuropsychology and other fields.

There is an association between damage to the ventromedial prefrontal cortex and a range of behaviors also common among persons with ASD.[43] These include inability to suppress emotions and impaired judgment and decision making. In a complex study of ToM among 49 individuals with brain lesions in prefrontal cortex and matched controls, Shamay-Tsoory and Aharon-Peretz[44] defined "cognitive" and "affective" ToM anatomic loci. In a related study, Kalbe and colleagues[45] disrupted right dorsolateral prefrontal cortical function using repetitive transcranial magnetic stimulation and then tested ToM. Both studies found functional independence of affective and cognitive ToM. These findings, if extended to functional deficits among persons with ASD, could aid expert witnesses in educating courts in matters that go beyond the typical boundaries of the simple cognitive standard of the M'Naghten Rule. This would have to be done with great caution, since there is evidence that deficits in the same areas of the brain may help explain impaired ToM among persons with psychopathy.[46]

Empathy deficits are often cited as a core feature of ASD. Although this may be true, it does not go far enough toward explaining the related deficits in information processing—both at a cognitive and an affective level.[47] Indeed, one can envision a legal argument for reduced culpability on the basis of lack of empathy per se backfiring, since empathy deficits are also seen in persons with antisocial and narcissistic personalities. Alongside the mentalizing circuitry are hormonal effects, for example, of oxytocin, which has long been known as a "prosocial" neuropeptide.[48] Oxytocin's wide-ranging effects on affiliative behaviors and inferring affective states of others[49] may be relevant to real deficits in the biologic substrate of violent behaviors.[50] At present, diagnostic testing of individual criminal defendants would not tend to include oxytocin, although peripheral measurements have been done.[51] Although meaningful connections between ASD and oxytocin are not clear enough for forensic purposes, interdisciplinary studies and therapeutic trials of oxytocin receptor agonists may shed light on them and could potentially inform offender dispositions.[52] Treatment options are especially welcome,[53] given the uncertainty of outcomes in autism and Asperger disorder.[54,55]

Criminal defendants with ASD who wish to use a defense based on mistake of fact may benefit from the literature on deficits in facial recognition and associated traits. Although not an invariable characteristic of persons with ASD,[56] it is a potential dynamic of aggressive behavior based on faulty processing of visual data. There is evidence that oxytocin increases memory for facial identity[57] and recognition of fear in another's face,[58] both in healthy persons.

CONCLUSIONS

There is little doubt that ASD is in the public consciousness, as evidenced by the increase in media coverage and scientific research. It would not be an exaggeration to cite the "Aspie" phenotype as a cultural meme, informally excusing awkwardness and nerdy behavior. There is even early evidence that the brain areas associated with ASD may give rise to enhanced creativity.[59] More important, there is now a robust autism advocacy movement, rooted in the concept of "neuro-diversity."[60] How this phenomenon translates into serious criminal cases remains to be seen. Although the small sampling of media and legal opinions reviewed here should not be taken as a definite indicator of trends, these facts show the many ways in which society is attempting to place the "square peg" of ASD into the "round hole" of criminal/juvenile justice. As Caruso (p. 538)[60] has recently observed, however, "autism's frontal attack on the notion of moral responsibility might prompt welcome reflections on the general ethics of retribution and punishment, but it also might boil down to empty sensationalism attached to a particular diagnostic label, without any systemic step forward in the communication between neuroscience and criminology."

Progress in the application of forensic psychiatry to the jurisprudence of criminal matters involving ASD will require a multipronged approach: education of police, teachers, health professionals, lawyers, and judges; refinements in our knowledge of the biology of ASD, sufficient to satisfy judicial gatekeepers; public awareness of behavioral differences, so that juries can fairly weigh evidence; and a revisiting of the standards for criminal responsibility. Decisions such as *Burr* in New Jersey may be a harbinger of a broadening of the types of evidence available to jurors and judges. The next step would be a legislative reform of the ancient cognitive test for "insanity," replacing it with a more realistic array of choices based on the science of human behavior.

REFERENCES

1. Bleuler E. *Dementia Praecox, or the Group of Schizophrenias [English translation]*. New York: International Universities Press; 1950.
2. Kanner L. Autistic disturbances of affective contact. *Nerv Child*. 1943; 2: 217–250.
3. Asperger H. Die autistischen psychopathen im Kindersalter. *Archiv fur Psychiatrie und Nervenkrankheiten*. 1944; 117: 76–136.
4. *Diagnostic and Statistical Manual of Mental Disorders: DSM-5*. Washington, DC: American Psychiatric Association; 2013.
5. www.dsm5.org/proposedrevision.aspx?rid=94# Accessed February 11, 2012.
6. Mouridsen SE. Current status of research on autism spectrum disorders and offending. *Res Autism Spectrum Dis*. 2012; 6(1): 79–86. doi:10.1016/j.rasd.2011.09.003.
7. Hingsburger D, Griffiths D, Quinsey V. Detecting counterfeit deviance: differentiating sexual deviance from sexual inappropriateness. *Habilitation Mental Health Care Newsletter*. 1991; 10: 51–54.
8. Mahoney M. Asperger's Syndrome and the Criminal Law: The Special Case of Child Pornography; 2009. Available from: www.harringtonmahoney.com. Accessed August 2, 2013.
9. Murphy W. *Orphan Diseases: New Hope for Rare Medical Conditions*. Brookfield, CT: Twenty-First Century Books; 2002.
10. Robison JE. *Raising Cubby: A Father and Son's Adventures with Asperger's, Trains, Tractors, and High Explosives*. New York: Crown Publishers; 2013.

11. Diverse City Press, Inc., Barrie, ON, Canada. http://www.diverse-city.com. Accessed August 4, 2013.
12. Debbaudt D. Autism risk and safety management. www.autismriskmanagement.com. Accessed August 4, 2013.
13. Mayer M. *Adam*. Fox Searchlight Films; 2009.
14. Tencer D. High school kid shot 5 times by SC police had autism: Report. October 18, 2009. Accessed at http://www.prisonplanet.com/high-school-kid-shot-5-times-by-sc-police-had-autism-report.html (link expired).
15. Osborn HE. Comment and casenote: what happened to "Paul's law"?: Insights on advocating for better training and better outcomes in encounters between law enforcement and persons with autism spectrum disorders. *University of Colorado Law Review*. 2008; 79: 333–379.
16. Ohio v. *Eal, Defendant-Appellant, 2012* Ohio 1373 (2012).
17. Robison JE. *Look Me in the Eye*. New York: Crown Publishers; 2007.
18. Allen D, Evans C, Hider A, Hawkins S, Peckett H, Morgan H. Offending behaviour in adults with Asperger syndrome. *J Autism Dev Disord*. 2008; 38: 748–758.
19. Schwartz-Watts DM. Asperger's disorder and murder. *J Am Acad Psychiatry Law*. 2005; 33: 390–393.
20. Sweet LJ. Odgren guilty as charged; Jury rejects insanity defense for killer. *Boston Globe*. April 30, 2010: 2.
21. Hammel L. *Judge rules against overturning Odgren life sentence in jail*. Telegram & Gazette (Massachusetts), September 16, 2010: B13.
22. Talbot J. *Seen and Heard: Supporting Vulnerable Children in the Youth Justice System*. London: Prison Reform Trust; 2010.
23. Hughes M. Hacker mentally ill since age of 17, says his mother. *Daily Telegraph* (London), March 18, 2011: 14.
24. Campbell D. Comment: An ignoble extradition: new clear evidence of hacker Gary McKinnon's Asperger's must persuade Parliament to protect him. *Guardian* (London), March 17, 2011: 38.
25. Murray J. Rock icon rescues hacker. *Sunday Express* (Scottish Edition), February 13, 2011: 10.
26. Slack J, Seamark M. 'I can't help you now': Mother's anger as Clegg 'washes his hands' of Gary McKinnon. *Daily Mail*, February 26, 2011. http://www.dailymail.co.uk/news/article-1360818/Clegg-washing-hands-Gary-tells-Mrs-McKinnon-help-son.html. Accessed August 3, 2013.
27. Wauhop B. Comment: Mindblindness: three nations approach the special case of the criminally accused individual with Asperger's Syndrome. *Penn State International Law Review*. 2009; 27: 959–991.
28. *U.S. v. Cottrell*, 333 Fed. Appx. 213 (2009).
29. *U.S. v. Anderson*, 68 M.J. 378 (2010).
30. *Missouri v. Boyd*, 143 S.W.3d (2004).
31. *Pearce v. Texas*, Court of Appeals of Texas, Fifth District, Dallas (2009).
32. *Commonwealth of Pennsylvania v. Daniel*, 597 Pa. 344; 951 A.2d 329 (2008).
33. *Florida v. Schoenwetter*, 46 So. 3d 535 (2010).
34. *State of New Jersey v. Burr*, 195 N.J. 119; 948 A.2d 627 (2008).
35. *State of New Jersey v. Burr*, 392 N.J. Super. 538, 921 A.2d 1135 (2007).
36. *California v. Larsen*, 205 Cal. App. 4th 810; 140 Cal. Rptr. 3d 762 (2012).
37. *Minnesota v. Anderson*, 789 N.W.2d 227 (2010).

38. *Minnesota v. Bouwman*, 328 N.W.2d 703, 705 (1982).

39. Haskins BG, Silva JA. Asperger's disorder and criminal behavior: forensic-psychiatric considerations. *J Am Acad Psychiatry Law.* 2006; 34: 374–384.

40. Baron-Cohen S. *Mindblindness: An Essay on Autism and Theory of Mind.* Cambridge, MA: MIT Press; 1995.

41. Hollander E, Kolevzon A, Coyle JT, eds. *Textbook of Autism Spectrum Disorders.* Washington, DC: American Psychiatric Press; 2011.

42. Silva JA. The relevance of neuroscience to forensic psychiatry. *J Am Acad Psychiatry Law.* 2009; 35: 6–9.

43. Bechara A. Editorial: The neurology of social cognition. *Brain.* 2002; 125: 1673–1675.

44. Shamay-Tsoory SG, Aharon-Peretz J. Dissociable prefrontal networks for cognitive and affective theory of mind: a lesion study. *Neuropsychologia.* 2007; 45: 3054–3067.

45. Kalbe E, Schlegel M, Sack AT, et al. Dissociating cognitive from affective theory of mind: a TMS study. *Cortex.* 2010; 46: 769–780.

46. Shamay-Tsoory SG, Harari H, Aharron-Peretz J, Levkovitz Y. The role of the orbitofrontal cortex in affective theory of mind deficits in criminal offenders with psychopathic tendencies. *Cortex.* 2010; 46: 668–677.

47. Decety J, Jackson PL. A social-neuroscience perspective on empathy. *Curr Directions Psychol Sci.* 2006; 15: 54–58.

48. Insel TR. Oxytocin—a neuropeptide for affiliation: evidence from behavioral, receptor autoradiographic, and comparative studies. *Psychoneuroendocrinology.* 1992; 17: 3–35.

49. Ross HE, Young LJ. Oxytocin and the neural mechanisms regulating social cognition and affiliative behavior. *Front Neuroendocrinol.* 2009; 30: 534–547.

50. Jolliffe D, Farrington DP. Empathy and offending: a systematic review and meta-analysis. *Aggression Viol Beh.* 2004; 9: 441–476.

51. Rubin LH, Carter CS, Drogos L, Pournajafi-Nazarloo H, Sweeney JA, Maki PM. Peripheral oxytocin is associated with reduced symptom severity in schizophrenia. *Schizo Res.* 2010; 124: 13–21.

52. Green JJ, Hollander E. Autism and oxytocin: new developments in translational approaches to therapeutics. *Neurotherapeutics.* 2010; 7: 250–257.

53. Andari E, Duhamel J-R, Zalla T, Herbrecht E, Leboyer M, Sirigu A. Promoting social behavior with oxytocin in high-functioning autism spectrum disorder. *Proc Nat Acad Sci USA.* 2010; 107: 4389–4394.

54. Cederlund M, Hagberg B, Billstedt E, Gillberg IC, Gillberg C. Asperger syndrome and autism: a comparative longitudinal follow-up study more than 5 years after original diagnosis. *J Autism Dev Disord.* 2008; 38: 72–85.

55. Tsatsanis KD. Outcome research in Asperger syndrome and autism. *Child Adolesc Psychiatr Cl North Am.* 2003; 12: 47–63.

56. Barton JJS, Cherasova MV, Hefter R, Cox TA, O'Connor M, Manoach DS. Are patients with social developmental disorders prosopagnosic? Perceptual heterogeneity in the Asperger and socio-emotional processing disorders. *Brain.* 2004; 127: 1706–1716.

57. Savaskan E, Ehrhardt R, Schulz, Walter M, Schachinger H. Post-learning intranasal oxytocin modulates human memory for facial identity. *Psychoneuroendocrinology.* 2008; 33: 368–374.

58. Fischer-Shofty M, Shamay-Tsoory SG, Harari H, Levkovitz Y. The effect of intranasal administration of oxytocin on fear recognition. *Neuropsychologia*. 2010; 48: 179–184.

59. Shamay-Tsoory, SG, Adler N, Aharon-Peretz J, Perry D, Mayseless N. The origins of originality: the neural bases of creative thinking and originality. *Neuropsychologia*. 2011; 49: 178–185.

60. Caruso D. Autism in the U.S.: social movement and legal change. *Am J Law Med*. 2010; 36: 483–539.

CHAPTER 6

Using fMRI for Lie Detection: Ready for Court?

OCTAVIO CHOI

In forensic settings, lying is a poison that wastes public resources and potentially corrupts justice. Although the adversarial court system in the United States was designed to compensate for biases and distortions inherent to each side, ascertaining matters of fact depends on the truthfulness of witnesses and the ability of fact finders to detect deception. Similarly, forensic psychiatrists' conclusions rely in part on behaviors and responses to questions—both of which can be faked. Forensic psychiatrists and judicial personnel are well aware that deception is common. The problem is that most people cannot accurately tell whether others are lying or telling the truth.[1-4]

Because of humans' limitations to detect deception, scientists have long searched for technological aids, for example the polygraph. However, the most recent of these technologies, functional magnetic resonance imaging (fMRI), offers a more direct approach to lie detection by peering into the liar's brain. Such technological advances are the culmination of the longstanding human quest to separate truth from lies. In ancient China, officials "placed dried rice in the mouths of criminal suspects, whom they told to spit out the grains. Suspects with rice still sticking on their tongues were exposed as liars" (p. 42).[5] Similarly, the Bedouins of Arabia "until quite recently required conflicting witnesses to lick a hot iron; the one whose tongue was burned was thought to be lying."[6] During the Spanish Inquisition, suspects "had to swallow a 'trial slice' of bread and cheese; if it stuck in the suspect's palate or throat, he or she was not telling the truth" (p. 767).[6] What do all these approaches have in common? Liars were assumed to be more anxious than truth tellers, and the increased sympathetic activation due to this resulted in reduced salivation.

Over time, scientists found increasingly precise ways to measure anxiety and other manifestations of autonomic arousal, which form the basis of the polygraph. With the advent of technologies that measure brain activity, such as electroencephalography (EEG) and fMRI, hopes for the development of accurate lie detection flourished. However, those hopes have yet to materialize, since no physiological "signature" dispositive for lying versus truth telling has yet been found. While the legal system has long confronted admissibility issues related to the polygraph since *Frye v. U.S.*[7] in 1923, challenges facing expert testimony regarding fMRI-based lie detection have only recently appeared in the courtroom. This chapter will review several questions regarding fMRI-based lie detection: (1) *How* does it work?; (2) How *well* does it work, and what are its limitations?; (3) Are results of fMRI-based lie detection studies *admissible* in court?; and (4) What are the ongoing legal concerns regarding lie detection technologies? First, a brief review of the history of functional neuroimaging.

A BRIEF HISTORY OF FUNCTIONAL NEUROIMAGING

The ability to noninvasively observe the activity of the human brain has been a sought-after dream for generations of neuroscientists. The great experimental physiologist Ivan Pavlov wrote in 1928: "If we could look through the skull into the brain of a consciously thinking person, and if the place of optimal excitability were luminous, then we should see playing over the cerebral surface, a bright spot with fantastic, waving borders constantly fluctuating in size and form, surrounded by a darkness more or less deep, covering the rest of the hemispheres" (p. 636).[8] With the advent of positron emission tomography (PET) in 1975, Pavlov's vision of activity-generated cerebral luminosity was realized. Later, the development of fMRI in the 1990s allowed neuroscientists to study the activity of the human brain in unprecedented detail, ushering in a new era of cognitive neuroscience.

PET scans are based on the principle that radionuclide tracers injected into the bloodstream concentrate in areas of increased neural activity. This is due to a phenomenon called *neurovascular coupling*, in which highly active areas of brain elicit an increase in localized blood supply, presumably to meet increased metabolic demands.[9] Depending on the radionuclide tracer used, different aspects of brain function can be measured and localized. However, PET scans suffer from several limitations, including poor spatial resolution and safety concerns related to the injection of radioactive materials.

The advent of fMRI has largely supplanted PET as a tool for investigations of brain activity, due to the fact that it can achieve high-resolution images without the need for radioactive tracers. Instead, fMRI works on the principle that hemoglobin in an oxygenated state has slightly different magnetic properties from hemoglobin in a deoxygenated state and thus can be discriminated by MRI. The relative proportions of oxygenated to deoxygenated hemoglobin are calculated and visualized as the BOLD (blood oxygenation level-dependent) signal. Because localized neural activity correlates tightly with blood flow, which in turn correlates with oxygenation levels, the BOLD signal can be a useful proxy indicator of brain activity.[10]

How accurately does the BOLD signal track neural activity? All correlations are imperfect, and several limitations have been pointed out by various researchers: (1) The correlation between neural activity and increased blood flow is sometimes imperfect, resulting in potential spatial and temporal mismatches between neuronal activity and vascular response; (2) Due to limits of spatial resolution, fMRI measures BOLD signals representing activity averaged across a significantly large population of neurons; and (3) Neurovascular coupling is still poorly understood, and the exact nature of the "neural activity" that elicits the vascular response is still unknown. At the current state of knowledge, the vascular response is thought to be elicited mostly by presynaptic activity of excitatory neurons; thus, BOLD signals may "miss" inhibitory activity in the brain.[11] However, within these limitations, the BOLD signal has proven itself over the past two decades of research to be a remarkably useful indicator of dynamic brain function.

fMRI-BASED DECEPTION TESTING

Sean Spence and his colleagues were the first to apply fMRI to elucidate neural activation patterns characteristic of lying versus truth telling.[12] Since then, refinements by neuroscientists such as Daniel Langleben and Andrew Kozel have produced fMRI-based predictive models that reportedly detect deception with accuracy rates up to 99%.[13,14]

Forward Inference, Reverse Inference

Early work in functional brain imaging established correlations between various mental tasks and resulting patterns of brain activation. For example, using PET scans, researchers were able to isolate areas in visual cortex activated by colored stimuli, which could be distinguished from areas activated by moving stimuli.[15] This is an example of *forward inference*, in which mental states are manipulated in the subject and resulting brain activation maps recorded. Subsequent studies established correspondences between a large variety of stimuli with unique resulting brain activation patterns. For example, using fMRI, a 1997 study identified a cortical area that appeared to be active only when faces were shown.[16] A subsequent study revealed a different cortical area that appeared to selectively respond when subjects were shown images of places, such as an outdoor scene, but not to other types of images, such as faces.[17]

Because faces and places evoke activity in distinct areas of cortex, researchers realized that in some cases, *reverse inference* could be possible. In regards to brain activity, reverse inference (also called "mind reading") is the process of analyzing brain activity and inferring the mental state that caused it. A study in 2000 demonstrated for the first time that analysis of a brain activation map allowed examiners to distinguish whether subjects were imagining a face or a place with high accuracy (85%).[18] With this study, fMRI-based mind reading was born.

The quest for a neural activity-based lie detector followed a similar course. The first wave of studies focused on the forward inference problem—establishing neural activation patterns correlated with lying versus truth telling. The second wave of studies then attempted to solve the reverse inference problem—looking at neural activation maps and making inferences about whether the subjects were lying or telling the truth.

The First Wave: Establishing Neural Correlates of Deception (Forward Inference)

Several problems are apparent when reviewing studies of brain activity correlated with deception. First, it is difficult to compare results from one study to another. This is partly due to the limitations of language in describing the complexity of the brain's anatomy. Different researchers sometimes use different names regarding the same anatomic brain area—one group's ventrolateral prefrontal cortex is another group's inferior temporal gyrus. The second problem in comparing studies has to do with the heterogeneity of lying paradigms. Lying is a complex phenomenon with "a hundred thousand shapes."[19] One expected result of this complexity is that different types of lying will generate different brain activity maps based on the different cognitive tasks that underlie its execution.

The third and perhaps most troubling problem is that collecting brain activity data using current technologies is a complex, multistep process that is not standardized between laboratories. In any given study, fMRI researchers must make decisions regarding the experimental paradigm, the image acquisition settings of the machine, adjustments to compensate for anatomic variations in individual brains, as well as other factors. The lack of imaging standards across labs is a well-known problem that has been pointed out by legal scholars[20] and judges.[21]

The fourth problem in interpreting functional imaging studies is that our functional understanding of brain areas is incomplete at best. Although it is clear that the brain accomplishes complex tasks in a distributed manner by invoking the activity of sets of cortical modules, it is unclear what any given cortical area "does," exactly. In some cases, it is relatively straightforward to ascribe meaningful functions to specific brain areas—this is especially true for well-defined perceptual areas such as visual cortex. Visual stimuli can be dissected into elementary components that are precisely defined by form, color, motion, and orientation, and all of these components are processed in anatomically well-defined cortical modules. In contrast, researchers lack a coherent ontology of cognition that could guide how to deconstruct complex tasks into elementary cognitive functions that are presumably processed by corresponding cortical modules.

Related to this is the problem of *reverse inference errors*. There are essentially an infinite number of potential stimuli that the brain must process with a limited number of cortical modules; thus, any given module will be used in a variety of tasks. Because of this, one cannot "know" what task the organism is engaged in simply by examining the activity of a particular cortical area. Ascribing specific functions to brain areas (i.e. "the activity in brain area Y means the subject was engaged in activity X") are thus prone to errors known as reverse inference errors.

Because of these problems, it makes little sense to become overly specific in ascribing a particular function to the activation of any particular brain area in a particular study. Rather, at our current state of knowledge, a better approach is to focus on broad patterns that emerge from the neuroimaging literature that converge with other lines of evidence regarding brain function, such as neuroanatomical lesion studies. That said, certain patterns of brain activity appear relatively consistently across many of the initial neuroimaging studies of deception. Broadly speaking, across a wide variety of lying paradigms, the prefrontal cortex is more active during lying versus truth telling. More specifically, various studies have reported increased activity in dorsolateral prefrontal cortex (DL-PFC),[22-27] ventrolateral prefrontal cortex (VL-PFC),[10,21,23,28,29] and anterior prefrontal cortex (aPFC).[19,21,24,25] Another area that is consistently reported to be more active during lying is the anterior cingulate cortex (ACC).[10,26,30,31]

The finding that areas of prefrontal cortex are involved in lying is consistent with what is known about the function of these areas from other lines of research. For example, from an evolutionary perspective, the emergence of skilled deception was a relatively late development, and correlates with the arrival and expansion of neocortex—of which prefrontal cortices were the most recent to appear.[32] From a developmental perspective, children do not start to lie until around the ages of 3 to 5, after language is acquired, consistent with the relatively later maturation of prefrontal cortex compared with parietal and temporal cortex.[33] The most recent confirmation of the importance of prefrontal cortex's role in deception comes from studies using transcranial direct current stimulation (tDCS). Various research groups have reported that tDCS applied over prefrontal cortex can alter the processing of deceptive responses, as measured by reaction times for deceptive answers to questions.[34-37] Studies of patients with prefrontal cortex lesions have established the prefrontal cortex as the seat of *executive functions*, which refers to a suite of cognitive skills needed for complex problem solving.[38] In fact, the descriptions of prefrontal lobe functions that emerge from lesion studies essentially amount to a description of the cognitive tasks required to lie. Lying is a kind of complex problem solving that involves generating a plausible, internally and externally consistent alternative while inhibiting the usual tendency (in most people) of telling the truth and inhibiting signs of autonomic arousal (guilt, anxiety, fear, excitement), while monitoring the response of the receiver and adjusting strategies in real time.

It should be noted that some of the increased brain activity associated with lying may be due to nonspecific arousal rather than deception-specific cognitive activity.[26] With regards to deception studies, a constant confounding variable that must be considered is physiologic arousal. Deceptive responses tend to be more anxiety producing than truthful responses; this is the basis of polygraph-aided lie detection. So how can we be sure that fMRI studies do not amount to anything more than a very expensive polygraph test? We can be reassured by careful investigations by Gamer and colleagues, who have examined this question using simultaneous measurements of galvanic skin conductance and fMRI during a guilty-knowledge paradigm of deception.[39,40] Their results demonstrate that much of the brain activity associated with deceptive responses correlates with arousal; however, after controlling for arousal, differential brain activity patterns for deception still persist. These results are consistent with other studies.[41]

The Second Wave: Constructing a Brain Activity-Based Lie Detector (Reverse Inference)

The first wave of studies helped elucidate neural correlates of deception at the group level. In those studies, brain activity maps of many individuals were collected during a deception task and averaged to produce a general map of brain activity thought to represent the brain at work while lying. Langleben and colleagues were the first group to take the next step: to create a lie detector that could perform reverse inference, one that could examine the brain activity of an individual and predict whether he or she was lying.[39] Using fMRI, the brain activity of 22 subjects was measured while they gave truthful and deceptive responses. The subjects were initially given two playing cards and told to deny possession of one card (lie) and acknowledge possession of the other (truth) when asked in the scanner. Activity maps pooling data from all subjects were combined to create a group-averaged map that highlighted areas of brain activity that appeared to differentiate lying from truth telling. Using the most promising areas of the group map in regards to whether subjects were lying or telling the truth, a model was constructed that predicted lying or truth telling depending on total brain activity in those areas. The model was then "tested" on 4 individuals who were not part of the model-building group. Based on individual brain scans, the model predicted lying with 76.5% accuracy.

Using a similar approach, Kozel and colleagues pooled brain activity from 30 individuals to construct a group map highlighting brain areas differentially active in lying versus truth telling.[12] A mock crime paradigm was used in which subjects "stole" one of two objects and were instructed to lie about it. Based on this group map, three brain areas were identified as informative in distinguishing lying from truth telling (ACC, OFC*, and DL-PFC) and were used to construct a predictive model. When tested on individuals not used to make the model, the model identified the "stolen" object with 90% accuracy. The study was replicated with 29 new individuals and achieved 86% accuracy.[42]

Even more impressive, Davatzikos and colleagues constructed a predictive lie-detection model using a radically different approach called *multivariate pattern analysis* (MVPA).[11] The MVPA approach involves training computers equipped with sophisticated learning algorithms to detect and classify patterns. In the "training" phase, the computer is fed brain activity maps and told whether each map represents lying or truth telling. Over time, using nonlinear machine learning algorithms, the computer "learns" to classify brain activity patterns as either more consistent with lying or with truth telling.[43] Using data from the same 22 individuals used to make the group averages in Langleben's model,[39] Davatzikos trained his MVPA classifier to the point where it achieved 99% accuracy when tested on those individuals. When the classifier was tested on individuals who were not part of the training set, it was able to perform at 88% accuracy, which was significantly more accurate than Langleben's model (76.5% accuracy).

MVPA models offer two significant advantages over the approaches taken by Langleben and Kozel, which are based on univariate analysis. Firstly, MVPA models are able to discern patterns of coordinated activity across the entire brain—patterns that would be too complex or subtle to detect by analyzing each brain area separately. As such, MVPA approaches have the potential to extract signal from the entire brain activity map. Secondly, MVPA models are nonlinear and can thus learn to classify highly divergent patterns of brain activity that correlate to lying or truth telling. This is very

---

* OFC refers to orbitofrontal cortex, which encompasses ventromedial and ventrolateral prefrontal cortex (VM-PFC and VL-PFC).

important, because deception-related brain activity is likely to vary across individuals and across different kinds of lies. In contrast, univariate models are based on pooled averages of brain activity and can thus only detect deception based on a convergent brain activity map. In essence, this is why Davatzikos's model was able to perform at 99% when tested on the individuals used to construct the model—the computer was able to "learn" the unique lying patterns for each individual. In contrast, univariate models misclassify individuals whose deception brain activity differs significantly from the pooled average—thus these models achieve lower levels of accuracy overall.

Since the publication of these papers, several companies have been established to commercialize fMRI lie detection. At this time, two attempts have been made to introduce testimony regarding fMRI lie detection in the trial phase of legal proceedings, both unsuccessfully: *Wilson v. Corestaff LP*[44] and *People v. Semrau*,[45] discussed below.

fMRI LIE DETECTION IN THE COURTROOM

Decisions regarding the admissibility of scientific expert testimony in the trial phase are determined by trial judges, who are guided by the applicable jurisdictional evidentiary standards. *Frye v. U.S.*[7] articulated a "general acceptance" standard under which scientific evidence should be admitted only if the science had "general acceptance in the particular field in which it belongs." The *Frye* standard was superseded in most jurisdictions by the Supreme Court's ruling in *Daubert v. Merrell Dow*,[46] which articulated a set of factors to help determine whether the proffered scientific evidence was reliable. These factors include inquiries regarding the testability, peer review, error rates, standards, and general scientific acceptance of the scientific technique in question. Because fMRI technology is so new, courts have been resistant to admitting results of fMRI studies. The only known case in which fMRI evidence (not regarding lie detection) has been allowed in court has been in the sentencing phase of a capital trial.

Brian Dugan, 2009

That case involved Brian Dugan, who had been convicted of murder in 2009 in Illinois.[47] In general, there are more permissible legal standards for the admission of evidence during the sentencing phase for capital crimes, in which courts typically allow "consideration of any relevant circumstances that could cause it to decline to impose the [death] penalty" (p. 317).[48] In Dugan's case, the trial court judge decided to disallow images of Dugan's fMRI brain scans but did allow expert testimony from Dr. Kent Kiehl regarding those scans. Dr. Kiehl testified that fMRI scans conducted on the defendant showed significant anomalies that indicated an organic basis of the defendant's psychopathy and should thus be considered a mitigating factor. After deliberation, the jury ultimately rejected arguments for mitigation, and Dugan received the death penalty. Although the jury ultimately rejected Dr. Kiehl's fMRI evidence, his testimony is thought have "turned it from a slam dunk for the prosecution into a much tougher case" (p. 342).[47] Dugan appealed this decision, but the appeal was dropped after Illinois abolished the death penalty in 2011.[49]

Wilson v. Corestaff Services LP (2010)

Wilson v. Corestaff Services was a sexual harassment lawsuit in which the plaintiff attempted to introduce results of fMRI "truth verification" testing conducted by Dr. Steven Laken to bolster the credibility of a key witness in her case. The case was based in New York, which follows the *Frye* standard. The trial court denied Wilson's request without an evidentiary hearing, based on the reasoning that the intended use of the fMRI evidence, to bolster the credibility of a witness, infringed on the traditional common-law view that "credibility is a matter solely for the jury. Anything that impinges on the province of the jury on issues of credibility should be treated with a great deal of skepticism" (p. 428).[44] Further, since credibility assessments were "within the ken of the average juror," expert testimony was improper and did not meet the so-called threshold requirement of the *Frye* standard. Finally, the court found that "even a cursory review of the scientific literature demonstrates that the plaintiff is unable to establish that the use of the fMRI test to determine truthfulness or deceit is accepted as reliable in the relevant scientific community" (p. 429),[44] thus failing a key prong of the *Frye* test.

People v. Semrau (2010)

In 2009, Lorne Semrau, a psychologist who ran several mental health clinics, was accused of fraudulently billing Medicare and Medicaid approximately $3 million in overcharges. Because the definition of fraud under federal statute requires that the actor conduct his actions *intentionally* and *knowingly*, the heart of the prosecution's case depended on Dr. Semrau's mental state at the time of his acts. Had he "*knowingly* devised a scheme or artifice to defraud a health care benefit program . . . and acted with the *intent* to defraud"? (p. 5)[45] Dr. Semrau hired Dr. Laken to determine whether fMRI tests could bolster his claims that his actions were "honest mistakes" based on a misunderstanding of governmental billing procedures.

Dr. Laken conducted scans on Dr. Semrau on two separate occasions. On the first occasion, Dr. Semrau was asked a set of questions regarding whether he knowingly used higher-reimbursing codes when he knew he should not. Based on analysis of fMRI activity during his responses, Dr. Laken concluded, "It appeared his brain showed he was telling the truth." Dr. Semrau was then asked a second set of questions regarding whether he knowingly incorrectly billed for services that should not have been separately billed. Dr. Laken concluded that for this second set of questions, "It appeared that he was lying when he said he was telling the truth."[50] After analyzing the data further, Dr. Laken proposed a new scanning session to revisit the second set of questions on the grounds that Dr. Semrau was fatigued during the second scan, which could have invalidated the results. A new scan was conducted on another day, focusing on the second set of questions. Dr. Laken concluded that this second scan indicated that Dr. Semrau was not being deceptive, and that "a finding such as this is 100% accurate in determining truthfulness from a truthful person" (p. 519).[21]

Because this was a federal case, the *Daubert* standard for the admissibility of scientific evidence applied. The *Daubert* standard requires scientific evidence to be *valid* and *relevant* to the issue at hand, with validity established by consideration of the so-called "*Daubert* factors." Unlike *Wilson*, the trial judge in this case, Judge Pham, conducted a full evidentiary hearing to evaluate whether Dr. Laken's fMRI evidence should be admitted. Judge Pham's reasoning in *Semrau* underlying his ultimate decision to exclude Dr. Laken's testimony serves as an excellent exposition of the shortcomings of fMRI lie detection in courtroom settings.

First, Judge Pham noted that fMRI lie detection appeared to meet the first two *Daubert* factors of testability and peer review. At the time of the decision, several published peer-reviewed articles existed that tested the ability of fMRI scans to detect deception, albeit in laboratory settings only. However, fMRI lie detection failed to fulfill the remaining *Daubert* factors regarding known error rates, standards for production of data, and general acceptance by the scientific community.

In terms of error rates, Judge Pham pointed out that although fMRI lie detection had been tested in a small number of people in controlled laboratory settings, it had not been tested in "real-life" settings, thus limiting its generalizability to "the real world." This is referred to as the *ecological validity problem*. It is perhaps the most serious problem of lie-detection technologies, preventing their use in the courtroom. Dr. Semrau was eventually convicted on three counts of healthcare fraud. He appealed this decision on the basis that evidence from his fMRI lie-detection testing should have been admitted. Semrau's request was denied and his conviction affirmed.[18]

Subjects chosen for laboratory studies of deception tend to be drawn from areas around the academic institution in which the studies are performed. Thus, subjects tend to be male, right-handed, young, well educated, healthy, and free of medications. They are then screened for medical, neurologic, and psychiatric illness and specifically excluded if significant conditions, including a history of drug abuse/dependence, are found. This is potentially a serious problem, because, as a whole, defendants in forensic settings may be quite different from the typical profile of subjects in lying studies, with high percentages of medical, neurologic, and psychiatric comorbidities reported.[51] These differences may translate into significantly different brain activation patterns when lying, thus limiting the applicability of findings from the lab.

Of specific concern in forensic settings, several studies have reported structural and functional brain differences in those with antisocial personality disorder, psychopaths, and pathological liars—differences that may result in significantly disparate brain-activation patterns when lying.[52-54] For example, Raine and colleagues have shown that those with antisocial personality disorder have reduced prefrontal gray matter volumes and reduced autonomic activity in response to stress.[50] Because many brain areas associated with deception may actually be detecting autonomic arousal,[37] those with reduced autonomic responses to lying would be expected to have brain activation patterns more consistent with truth telling.

This was confirmed recently in a fascinating study in which subjects were recruited from local university sports teams and were measured on various psychopathic personality traits using the Psychopathic Personality Inventory (a standard measure). Brain activity patterns were recorded in a deception task and increased activation was seen in VL-PFC, consistent with other deception studies. Additionally, the degree of activation was found to correlate *inversely* with the degree of psychopathy. That is, subjects who were more psychopathic had brain patterns when lying that more resembled truth telling.[55]

Literature on the development of expertise has noted that long-term practice can drive structural change in the brain.[56,57] Considering that pathological liars have considerably more practice in deceiving others than nonpathological liars, the question arises whether they may have structural brain differences in areas associated with deception. This question has been answered by recent structural MRI studies, which report that pathological liars have significantly more white matter in prefrontal cortex than the other groups.[51,52] One interpretation of these results is that by long-term practice, pathological liars have increased white matter of areas important in lying. The other is that they were genetically endowed with more white matter in these areas, which gifted them with a facility for deception. Ultimately, these findings may be due to reinforcing effects of both genetic endowment and practice.

Do these structural differences result in brains that are "more efficient" in lying compared with novice liars? A preliminary study by Jiang and colleagues indicates that they do.[58] They found that degree of activation in DL-PFC and ACC with deceptive responses correlated inversely with deceptive capabilities. That is, more accomplished liars showed less activation in those areas and resembled brain patterns more consistent with truth telling in normal controls. In addition to long-term structural changes induced by practice over weeks to months, many researchers have reported dramatic functional differences in brain activity induced by practice over very short periods of time, over a time course of minutes.[59-61] Taken as a sum, these studies underscore the complexities inherent in drawing conclusions from measures of brain activity in individuals.

Finally, no discussion of lie-detection validity is complete without a mention of possible countermeasures. The first paper has emerged regarding countermeasures used in fMRI lie detection, and it is concerning.[62] In that study a MVPA classifier was used that, when tested on new subjects, performed at 100% accuracy in detecting when subjects were lying. The subjects were then taught a simple countermeasure of making a specific wiggling action with their fingers when responding. When rescanned with this instruction, the MVPA classifier's performance dropped from 100% accuracy to 33% accuracy. Over time, refinement of lie-detection algorithms may be able to overcome particular countermeasures, but of course, other countermeasures can be invented in response, creating a perpetual cat-and-mouse game between liars and lie detectors.

Thus far, we have discussed ecological validity concerns regarding the fact that subjects studied in the lab may be quite different from "real-world" forensic populations. Another source of ecological validity problems is the fact that the *types of lies* studied in the lab are quite different than the types of lies told in forensic settings. Paradigms for deception in the lab are highly simplistic (for example, denying the possession of a playing card), are typically low stakes (no punishment for failing to lie effectively), and are artificial in that subjects are directed to lie by the research team. Obviously, these are conditions that are quite different from "real-world" lying in forensic settings, which tend to be high stakes and in which the liar freely chooses to lie. The heterogeneity of types of lying (omission v. commission, low stakes v. high stakes, compliance v. defiance, memorized v. spontaneous) is dauntingly large, and since each type of lie may generate unique profiles of brain activation, they may have to be individually validated.

Another concern was raised in *Semrau* regarding the timing of fMRI testing. Unlike research studies, in which subjects are typically questioned about events that took place immediately prior to the scan, Dr. Semrau was questioned about events that occurred 6 to 8 years prior to his scans. Judge Pham noted that these large temporal differences limited the validity of interpretations of Dr. Semrau's test results on the basis of lab studies.

In summary, because of differences in subject population, lying paradigm, and timing of testing, Judge Pham correctly concluded that Dr. Laken's testimony did not satisfy *Daubert* standards regarding ecological validity. In addition, Judge Pham noted that fMRI lie detection suffered from a lack of standardization that further limited its validity: "Because the use of fMRI-based lie detection is still in its early stages of development, standards controlling the real-life application have not yet been established. Without such standards, a court cannot adequately evaluate the reliability of a particular lie detection examination" (p. 31).[45]

LIE DETECTION: A LEGAL PERSPECTIVE

In general, many courts have expressed deep reservations regarding the admission of lie-detection studies dating back to *Frye* in 1923. Many, as in *Semrau*, have found the underlying scientific technologies unsound and have thus denied admission based on *Frye* or *Daubert* criteria. Others have asserted that lie-detection evidence should be excluded on the basis that it is more prejudicial than probative. Still others cite concerns that testimony regarding lie detection usurps the traditional role of the jury as the ultimate arbiter of credibility. Each of these arguments regarding reliability, prejudice, and the jury's proper role as bases to exclude evidence has vigorous critics, resulting in a confusing legal landscape full of divergent opinions.

Considerations of prejudice and probity relate to fears that certain kinds of information will render jurors irrational. In the case of brain imaging evidence, some studies suggest that people can be swayed by arguments that are accompanied with brain images,[63,64] even if the images do not add any "real" information.[65,66] In this view, brain images are "seductive" because they are visually compelling and carry the imprimatur of "big science." However, it should be noted that the largest and most recent study regarding the impact of neuroimages on jurors' decision making found "a lack of any impact of neuroimages on the decisions of our mock jurors" (p. 382).[67] With regards to polygraph evidence, Justice Clarence Thomas stated in his majority opinion in *Scheffer*[68] that "jurisdictions...may legitimately be concerned about the risk that juries will give excessive weight to the opinions of a polygrapher, clothed as they are in scientific expertise...Such jurisdictions may legitimately determine that the aura of infallibility attending polygraph evidence can lead jurors to abandon their duty to assess credibility and guilt" (p. 314).[68]

Critics of such reasoning counter that prejudicial concerns are overstated and that juries have shown themselves capable of evaluating complex scientific evidence.[69] As such, they urge a more lenient threshold for the admission of scientific evidence—even for evidence that is potentially unreliable and confusing. In fact, the *Daubert* court's stated motive in expanding the *Frye* standard was to embrace a "general approach of relaxing the traditional barriers to opinion testimony" (p. 588),[46] an approach that trusted jurors' ability to determine the quality of evidence through the adversarial process: "Vigorous cross-examination, presentation of contrary evidence, and careful instruction on the burden of proof are the traditional and appropriate means of attacking shaky but admissible evidence" (p. 596).[46]

Resistance to the admission of lie-detection evidence is often clothed under the argument that lie detection infringes on the jury's role in assessing credibility. Perhaps the most cited advocate for this line of reasoning is Justice Clarence Thomas, who wrote, regarding the role of polygraph testing in *Scheffer*: "A fundamental premise of our criminal trial system is that 'the jury is the lie detector'. Determining the weight and credibility of witness testimony, therefore, has long been held to be the 'part of every case [that] belongs to the jury, who are presumed to be fitted for it by their natural intelligence and their practical knowledge of men and the ways of men'. By its very nature, polygraph evidence may diminish the jury's role in making credibility determinations" (p. 313).[68]

According to Justice Thomas, lie-detection evidence is not only prejudicial but also unnecessary because average jurors are "fitted for it [detecting deception] by their natural intelligence and their practical knowledge"—and perhaps we are. The capacity to deceive others stems from the same neural machinery that evolved to allow us to understand what others are thinking—an ability which presumably conferred survival advantages by facilitating cooperation between individuals.[70] Thus, our ability to lie likely coevolved with our ability to detect deception, and we do it all the time. However, being "naturally fitted" to judge deception does not mean we are good at it. In fact, the uncomfortable truth is that most people perform barely above chance levels in discriminating truth from lie.[71,72] There is a profound disconnect between how good people *think* they are at detecting deception and their actual ability to do so.[68] In contrast, fMRI methods are approaching 99% accuracy in detecting lies, albeit under controlled laboratory conditions. As lie detectors improve, it will increasingly call into question the premise that people cannot be aided in their credibility determinations by technology.

REFERENCES

1. Ekman P, O'Sullivan M. Who can catch a liar? *Am Psychol*. 1991; 46: 913–920.
2. Kraut R, Poe D. On the line: the deception judgements of customs inspectors and laymen. *J Pers Soc Psychol*. 1980; 39: 784–798.

3. DePaulo BMK, Kashy DA, Kirkendol SE, Wyer MM. Lying in everyday life. *J Pers Soc Psychol*. 1996; 70: 979–995.

4. Vrij A. Why professionals fail to catch liars and how they can improve. *Legal Criminol Psychol*. 2004; 9: 159–181.

5. Schafer E. Ancient science and forensics. In: Embar-Seddon A, Pass AD, eds. *Forensic Science*. Salem, MA: Salem Press; 2008: 40–43.

6. Kleinmuntz B, Szucko JJ. Lie detection in ancient and modern times: a call for contemporary scientific study. *Am Psychol*. 1984; 39: 766–776.

7. *Frye* v. *United States*, 293 F. 1013 (D.C. Cir. 1923).

8. Brugger P. Pavlov on neuroimaging. *J Neurol Neurosurg Psychiatry*. 1997; 62: 636.

9. Raichle ME. Functional neuroimaging: a historical and physiological perspective. In: Cabeza R, Kingstone A, eds. *Handbook of Functional Neuroimaging of Cognition*. Cambridge, MA: MIT Press; 2006: 3–20.

10. Ogawa S, Lee TM, Kay AR, Tank DW. Brain magnetic resonance imaging with contrast dependent on blood oxygenation. *Proc Natl Acad Sci USA*. 1990; 87: 9868–9872.

11. Logothetis NK. What we can do and what we cannot do with fMRI. *Nature*. 2008; 453: 869–878.

12. Spence SA, Farrow TF, Herford AE, Wilkinson ID, Zheng Y, Woodruff PW. Behavioural and functional anatomical correlates of deception in humans. *Neuroreport*. 2001; 12: 2849–2853.

13. Davatzikos C, Ruparel K, Fan Y, et al. Classifying spatial patterns of brain activity with machine learning methods: application to lie detection. *NeuroImage*. 2005; 28: 663–668.

14. Kozel FA, Johnson KA, Mu Q, Grenesko EL, Laken SJ, George MS. Detecting deception using functional magnetic resonance imaging. *Biol Psych*. 2005; 58: 605–613.

15. Zeki S, Watson JD, Lueck CJ, Friston KJ, Kennard C, Frackowiak RS. A direct demonstration of functional specialization in human visual cortex. *J Neurosci*. 1991; 11: 641–649.

16. Kanwisher N, McDermott J, Chun MM. The fusiform face area: a module in human extrastriate cortex specialized for face perception. *J Neurosci*. 1997; 17: 4302–4311.

17. Epstein R, Kanwisher N. A cortical representation of the local visual environment. *Nature*. 1998; 392: 598–601.

18. O'Craven KM, Kanwisher N. Mental imagery of faces and places activates corresponding stimulus-specific brain regions. *J Cog Neurosci*. 2000; 12: 1013–1023.

19. Montaigne M. *The Complete Essays of Montaigne*. Stanford: Stanford University Press; 1958: 24.

20. Brown T, Murphy E. Through a scanner darkly: functional neuroimaging as evidence of a criminal defendant's past mental states. *Stanford Law Review*. 2010; 62: 1119–1208.

21. *United States* v. *Semrau*, 693 F.3d 510 (6th Cir. 2012).

22. Lee TM, Liu HL, Tan LH, et al. Lie detection by functional magnetic resonance imaging. *Human Brain Mapping*. 2002; 15: 157–164.

23. Ganis G, Kosslyn SM, Stose S, Thompson WL, Yurgelun-Todd DA. Neural correlates of different types of deception: an fMRI investigation. *Cerebral Cortex*. 2003; 13: 830–836.

24. Nuñez JM, Casey BJ, Egner T, Hare T, Hirsch J. Intentional false respond-ing shares neural substrates with response conflict and cognitive control. *NeuroImage*. 2005; 25: 267–277.

25. Phan KL, Magalhaes A, Ziemlewicz TJ, Fitzgerald DA, Green C, Smith W. Neural correlates of telling lies: a functional magnetic resonance imaging study at 4 Tesla. *Acad Radiol*. 2005; 12: 164–172.

26. Abe N, Suzuki M, Mori E, Itoh M, Fujii T. Deceiving others: distinct neural responses of the prefrontal cortex and amygdala in simple fabrication and deception with social interaction. *J Cog Neurosci*. 2007; 19: 287–295.

27. Abe N, Fujii T, Hirayama K, et al. Do parkinsonian patients have trouble telling lies? The neurobiological basis of deceptive behaviour. *Brain*. 2009; 132: 1386–1395.

28. Kozel FA, Revell LJ, Lorberbaum JP, et al. A pilot study of functional mag-netic resonance imaging brain correlates of deception in healthy young men. *J Neuropsych Clin Neurosci*. 2004; 16: 295–305.

29. Spence SA, Hunter MD, Farrow TF, et al. A cognitive neurobiological account of deception: evidence from functional neuroimaging. *Phil Trans Royal Soc London Series B Biol Sci*. 2004; 359: 1755–1762.

30. Langleben DD, Schroeder L, Maldjian JA, et al. Brain activity during simulated deception: an event-related functional magnetic resonance study. *NeuroImage*. 2002; 15: 727–732.

31. Lee TM, Liu HL, Chan CC, Ng YB, Fox PT, Gao JH. Neural correlates of feigned memory impairment. *NeuroImage*. 2005; 28: 305–313.

32. Teffer K, Semendeferi K. Human prefrontal cortex: evolution, development, and pathology. *Prog Brain Res*. 2012; 195: 191–218.

33. Casey BJ, Tottenham N, Liston C, Durston S. Imaging the developing brain: what have we learned about cognitive development? *Trends Cog Sci*. 2005; 9: 104–110.

34. Priori A, Mameli F, Cogiamanian F, et al. Lie-specific involvement of dorsolat-eral prefrontal cortex in deception. *Cerebral Cortex*. 2008; 18: 451–455.

35. Mameli F, Mrakic-Sposta S, Vergari M, et al. Dorsolateral prefrontal cortex specifically processes general—but not personal—knowledge deception: mul-tiple brain networks for lying. *Behav Brain Res*. 2010; 211: 164–168.

36. Karim AA, Schneider M, Lotze M, et al. The truth about lying: inhibition of the anterior prefrontal cortex improves deceptive behavior. *Cerebral Cortex*. 2010; 20: 205–213.

37. Fecteau S, Boggio P, Fregni F, Pascual-Leone A. Modulation of untruthful responses with non-invasive brain stimulation. *Front Psych*. 2012; 3: 97.

38. Cummings JL, Mega MS. *Neuropsychiatry and Behavioral Neuroscience*. New York: Oxford University Press; 2003.

39. Gamer M, Bauermann T, Stoeter P, Vossel G. Covariations among fMRI, skin conductance, and behavioral data during processing of concealed information. *Human Brain Mapping*. 2007; 28: 1287–1301.

40. Gamer M, Klimecki O, Bauermann T, Stoeter P, Vossel G. fMRI-activation pat-terns in the detection of concealed information rely on memory-related effects. *Soc Cog Affect Neurosci*. 2012; 7(5): 506–515.

41. Langleben DD, Loughead JW, Bilker WB, et al. Telling truth from lie in indi-vidual subjects with fast event-related fMRI. *Human Brain Mapping*. 2005; 26: 262–272.

42. Kozel FA, Johnson KA, Grenesko EL, et al. Functional MRI detection of deception after committing a mock sabotage crime. *J Foren Sci*. 2009; 54: 220–231.

43. Haxby JV. Multivariate pattern analysis of fMRI: the early beginnings. *NeuroImage*. 2012; 62: 852–855.

44. *Wilson* v. *Corestaff Services*, 28 Misc. 3d 425, 900 N.Y.S.2d 639 (N.Y. Sup. Ct. 2010).

45. *United States* v. *Semrau*, No. 07-10074 (W.D Tenn. May 31, 2010).

46. *Daubert* v. *Merrell Dow Pharmaceuticals, Inc.*, 509 U.S. 579 (1993).

47. Hughes V. Science in court: head case. *Nature*. 2010; 464: 340–342.

48. *Penry* v. *Lynaugh*. 492 U.S. 302 (1989).

49. Langleben DD, Moriarty JC. Using brain imaging for lie detection: where science, law and research policy collide. *Psychol Pub Pol Law*. 2012; 19: 222–234.

50. Shen FX, Jones OD. Brain scans as evidence: truths, proofs, lies, and lessons. *Mercer Law Review*. 2011; 62: 861–883.

51. James DJ, Glaze LE. *Mental Health Problems of Prison and Jail Inmates*. Washington, DC: US Department of Justice, Office of Justice Programs, Bureau of Justice Statistics; 2006.

52. Raine A, Lencz T, Bihrle S, LaCasse L, Colletti P. Reduced prefrontal gray matter volume and reduced autonomic activity in antisocial personality disorder. *Arch Gen Psych*. 2000; 57: 119–127.

53. Yang Y, Raine A, Lencz T, Bihrle S, Lacasse L, Colletti P. Prefrontal white matter in pathological liars. *Br J Psych*. 2005; 187: 320–325.

54. Yang Y, Raine A, Narr KL, et al. Localisation of increased prefrontal white matter in pathological liars. *Br J Psych*. 2007; 190: 174–175.

55. Fullam RS, McKie S, Dolan MC. Psychopathic traits and deception: functional magnetic resonance imaging study. *Br J Psych*. 2009; 194: 229–235.

56. Draganski B, Gaser C, Kempermann G, et al. Temporal and spatial dynamics of brain structure changes during extensive learning. *J Neurosci*. 2006; 26: 6314–6317.

57. Schlaug G, Forgeard M, Zhu L, Norton A, Norton A, Winner E. Training-induced neuroplasticity in young children. *Ann NY Acad Sci*. 2009; 1169: 205–208.

58. Jiang W, Liu H, Liao J, et al. A functional MRI study of deception among offenders with antisocial personality disorders. *Neuroscience*. 2013; 244: 90–98.

59. Raichle ME. Behind the scenes of functional brain imaging: a historical and physiological perspective. *Proc Natl Acad Sci USA*. 1998; 95: 765–772.

60. Milham MP, Banich MT, Claus ED, Cohen NJ. Practice-related effects demonstrate complementary roles of anterior cingulate and prefrontal cortices in attentional control. *NeuroImage*. 2003; 18: 483–493.

61. Phelps EA. Lying outside the laboratory: the impact of imagery and emotion on the neural circuitry of lie detection. In: Bizzi E, Hyman SE, Raichle ME, et al., eds. *Using Imaging to Identify Deceit: Scientific and Ethical Questions*. Cambridge, MA: American Academy of Arts and Sciences; 2009: 14–22.

62. Ganis G, Rosenfeld JP, Meixner J, Kievit RA, Schendan HE. Lying in the scanner: covert countermeasures disrupt deception detection by functional magnetic resonance imaging. *NeuroImage*. 2011; 55: 312–319.

63. Gurley JR, Marcus DK. The effects of neuroimaging and brain injury on insanity defenses. *Behav Sci Law*. 2008; 26: 85–97.

64. Greene E, Cahill BS. Effects of neuroimaging evidence on mock juror decision making. *Behav Sci Law*. 2012; 30: 280–296.

65. McCabe DP, Castel AD. Seeing is believing: the effect of brain images on judgments of scientific reasoning. *Cognition*. 2008; 107: 343–352.

66. Weisberg DS, Keil FC, Goodstein J, Rawson E, Gray JR. The seductive allure of neuroscience explanations. *J Cog Neurosci*. 2008; 20(3): 470–477.

67. Schweitzer NJ, Saks MJ, Murphy ER, Roskies AL, Sinnott-Armstrong W, Gaudet LM. Neuroimages as evidence in a *mens rea* defense: no impact. *Psychol Pub Pol Law*. 2011; 17: 357–393.

68. *U.S.* v. *Scheffer*, 523 U.S. 303 (1998).

69. Nance DA, Morris SB. Juror understanding of DNA evidence: an empirical assessment of presentation formats for trace evidence with a relatively small random-match probability. *J Leg Stud*. 2005; 34: 395–444.

70. Byrne RW, Corp N. Neocortex size predicts deception rate in primates. *Proc Royal Soc London B Biol Sci*. 2004; 271: 1693–1699.

71. Ekman P, O'Sullivan M, Friesen W, Scherer K. Face, voice, and body in detecting deceit. *J Nonverbal Behav*. 1991; 15: 125–135.

72. Ekman P, O'Sullivan M, Frank MG. A few can catch a liar. *Psychol Sci*. 1999; 10: 263–266.

CHAPTER 7

Sleep Disorders and Criminal Responsibility

CLARENCE WATSON, MARK R. PRESSMAN, AND
KENNETH J. WEISS*

"A great perturbation in nature, to receive at once the benefit of sleep, and do the effects of watching!"[1] This commentary by Shakespeare's physician character in *Macbeth* speaks to the paradoxical phenomenon of sleepwalking, as he observes a sleeping Lady Macbeth confess to her prior bad acts. While there may be little argument that a sleeping person who confesses to prior crimes might be held responsible for those crimes, a different predicament has generated debate over the centuries: What is to be made of the person whose bad acts occur during sleep?

Historically, the view of sleep and behavior has been epitomized in the saying *In somno voluntas non erat libera* (A sleeping person has no free will). How should a person who engages in a seemingly criminal act during sleep be held responsible? For centuries, somnambulism and related phenomena had been considered supernatural, until psychoanalytic theory attempted to give dream-states meaning related to prior psychological trauma.[2] Only in 1953 was rapid eye movement (REM) sleep described as a separate state of consciousness. In 1964, the first studies of sleepwalking and sleep terrors in a modern sleep laboratory were conducted. These studies resulted in the surprising conclusion that sleepwalking was not a REM-sleep-related

* Portions of this chapter were previously published as: Weiss KJ, Watson C, Markov D, del Busto E, Foubister N, Doghramji K. Parasomnias, violence and the law. *J Psychiatry Law.* 2011; 39: 249–286. Used with permission from Federal Legal Publications, Inc., Somers, NY.

phenomenon, thus dispelling psychoanalytic dream/psychological trauma interpretations of sleepwalking.

Bonkalo was the first to collect a series of cases of putative disorders of arousal associated with criminal acts and adjudicated in court.[3] He recounted a 1791 criminal case in Silesia where a man killed his wife with an axe during his sleep. The defense argued that the defendant was not fully awake at the time of the killing, which occurred during "sleep drunkenness" (*Schlaftrunkenheit*). It was argued, in keeping with the above Latin aphorism, that the defendant was (legally) asleep when he acted and had "no free will" to commit the crime. The German literature, according to Bonkalo, includes about 20 such cases; in French the episodes are termed *l'ivresse du sommeil*.

When Dr. Benjamin Rush wrote about somnambulism and "incubus" (nightmare) in the early 19th century, there was the emerging view that their physiology could be known.[4] He likened dreaming and somnambulism to paroxysmal delirium, relating them to diseased blood vessels in the brain. Isaac Ray, the father of American forensic psychiatry, did not believe that an individual should be held criminally responsible for behaviors occurring during sleep. In his chapter in *A Treatise on the Medical Jurisprudence of Insanity*[5] "Legal Consequences of Somnambulism," Ray stated, "As a somnambulist does not enjoy the free and rational exercise of his understanding, and is more or less unconscious of his outward relations, none of his acts during the paroxysms, can rightfully be imputed to him as crimes."[5,p415] Writing from the point of view of a skeptical forensic psychiatrist, Ray also acknowledged *somnolentia* and *somnambulism* as worthy of consideration in questions of criminal responsibility, but he was quick to add a chapter on "simulated somnambulism." Despite these concerns, when sleepwalking was proved in court in the 19th century, there was often an acquittal or "special verdict."

Even before scientists studied sleep physiology, society considered it self-evident that sleeping persons would not be criminally responsible. Although the problem of malingering was acknowledged in early American forensic psychiatry, the defendant with sleepwalking or sleep drunkenness was treated leniently. Over the past half-century, sleep physiology has been examined, and there is a developing nomenclature for sleep disorders. Although there is no clear-cut correlation between violence and sleep, parasomnias have been implicated. Violent behavior during sleep is a rare occurrence with troubling implications for adjudicating criminal responsibility. In this chapter, we discuss the scientific understanding of parasomnias and the jurisprudence of violent behavior during sleep. We will focus on the nexus between sleep pathology and the capacity to form criminal intent—a matter that has interested scientists and the public for hundreds of years.

Parasomnias, defined as undesirable behavioral, physiological, or experiential events that accompany sleep, are common in the general population.[6] Box 7.1 lists differential diagnoses to consider during clinical evaluations of sleep-related behaviors. The nomenclature and classification of parasomnias have undergone refinements as knowledge of sleep physiology has improved. The *Diagnostic and Statistical Manual of Mental Disorders, 2nd Edition (DSM-II)*,[7] barely acknowledged sleep pathology as a "special symptom," and *DSM-III*[8] noted childhood disorders (sleepwalking and sleep terror). The *DSM-III-R*[9] classified the new "parasomnias" under sleep disorders, distinguishing nightmare disorder, sleep terror disorder, and sleepwalking disorder, and *DSM-IV*[10] and *DSM-IV-TR*[11] continued to list these as well as REM-sleep behavior disorder (in the "not otherwise specified" category). The latest classifications come from the *DSM-5*[12] and the system developed by the American Academy of Sleep Medicine in the recently published *International Classification of Sleep Disorders (ICSD-3)*.[13] Both of these recently published classification systems are notable for changes in the role of alcohol as a trigger. In *DSM-IV* and *ICSD-2*, alcohol was listed as a potential trigger for disorders of arousal.[10,14] In the current versions of these classification systems this view has been deleted (*DSM-5*) or it has been clearly stated that disorders of arousal may not be diagnosed in the presence of alcohol (*ICSD-3*).

Box 7.1: DIFFERENTIAL DIAGNOSIS FOR SLEEP-RELATED BEHAVIORS

Disorders of arousal
   Confusional arousal
      Sexual behavior in sleep
   Sleepwalking
      Sleep driving
   Sleep terrors
   Sleep eating
REM-sleep behavior disorder
Nightmares
Nocturnal seizures
Hypnogogic/hypnopompic hallucinations
Somniloquy
Dissociative states
PTSD
Malingering

Parasomnias, as a rule, occur more frequently in children than in adults, with the exception of REM-sleep behavior disorder, which is more common in men over 50. The most common parasomnias occur during deep sleep and follow a sudden arousal. These disorders are most often called disorders of arousal and include confusional arousals, sleep terrors, and sleepwalking. Recent neuroimaging studies suggest that disorders of arousal are secondary to brain state dissociation. These disorders are characterized by a profound loss of higher cognitive function, including memory, planning, and attention. Disorders of arousal most frequently follow prior acute sleep deprivation and situational stress. Violent behavior during sleep is rare but may occur if the sleeper is provoked by or in close proximity to others.

We present the following summary of parasomnias in adults and children, followed by a discussion of sexual behavior during sleep, to aid expert witnesses who may be called upon to explain sleep-related violence to a judge or jury.

SLEEP-STAGE CORRELATIONS

Sleep consists of two strikingly different states, REM sleep and non-REM (NREM) sleep, which alternate in a cyclical fashion. Sleep begins with a "shallow" stage N1 of NREM and "deepens" to NREM stages N2 and N3, which are followed by the first brief episode of REM after approximately 90 minutes. After the first sleep cycle, NREM and REM sleep continue alternating in a cyclical fashion, approximately 90 minutes per complete cycle. Stage N3 of NREM sleep (also known as deep sleep, delta sleep, or slow-wave sleep) predominates during the first third of the night. REM-sleep episodes become longer as the night progresses, and the longest REM periods are found during the last third of the night.[15]

Parasomnias can arise from any stage of sleep (REM and NREM) or sleep–wake transitions and are classified into distinct syndromes on this basis. Disorders of arousal, for example, are the most prevalent of the NREM parasomnias. Typically, they occur during the first third of the night, when deep (NREM) sleep is most abundant. REM-sleep parasomnias are more likely to emerge during the latter portion of the sleep period, when REM sleep is most abundant. Upon awakening from REM parasomnias, individuals are typically alert and have vivid recollection of dream content and mental activity. In contrast, individuals with NREM parasomnias who are awakened are typically disoriented and confused. Recent reports suggest that sleep terrors and sleepwalking may be associated with recall of dreamlike mentation. However, as compared to the typically hallucinatory content of REM dreaming, NREM mentation most often involves a single static image that may be frightening (e.g., house on fire, intruder in bedroom). However, they have no recollection of their actual behavior in the real world.

NREM PARASOMNIAS: DISORDERS OF AROUSAL AND SLEEP–WAKE TRANSITION DISORDERS

Disorders of arousal include confusional arousals, sleep terrors, and sleepwalking. These parasomnias are best conceptualized as partial or incomplete arousals from deep sleep. During these events, states of sleep and wakefulness coexist and are intermixed. The sleeper is in a state between deep sleep and full wakefulness—partially asleep and partially awake.[16-18] This may also relate to certain parts of the brain that remain active while other parts of the brain are deactivated.[19]

Disorders of arousal are common phenomena in childhood and become less prevalent after age 5.[20-24] Generally, a family history of disorders of arousal predisposes the patient to these parasomnias.[25] Episodes of confusional arousal, sleep terror, or sleepwalking may be facilitated by factors that deepen sleep, such as young age, the use of central nervous system (CNS) depressants, recovery from sleep deprivation, or fever. While alcohol is considered a CNS depressant and results in nocturnal wandering, alcohol is no longer considered to be a triggering factor for sleepwalking. Factors that disrupt sleep and introduce arousals into the normal sleep process, such as pain, touch, environmental noises, periodic limb movements, sleep apneas, and full bladder, can also trigger disorders of arousal.[16]

Confusional Arousals

Confusional arousals result from partial or incomplete arousal from deep (NREM) sleep, typically during the first third of the night. They are identical in most respects to sleepwalking but only occur with the sleeper in bed. When the sleeper leaves the bed, the behavior is considered to be sleepwalking. Their prevalence in the 15- to 24-year-old population is 6%; in those over age 65 it is 1%.[26] Confusional arousals are manifested by episodes of confused and slowed thinking, disorientation to time and place, perceptual impairment, and inappropriate responsiveness to external stimuli. Complex motor activity is absent, but individuals may exhibit automatic behaviors, such as picking at clothes and linens, kicking, thrashing in bed, and using objects inappropriately. Episodes typically last from seconds to minutes and are usually followed by retrograde amnesia for the event.[14,18,25] These phenomena may result in cognitive abnormalities; for example, sleep-deprived physicians who are suddenly awakened from deep sleep may experience confusional arousals and may be at increased risk for judgment and decision errors.

Sleep Terrors (*Pavor Nocturnus*, Incubus Attacks)

Sleep terror attacks arise abruptly, usually during the first third of the night. The child or adult sits up with an expression of terror, emits a piercing scream, and appears frightened. The individual usually displays autonomic arousal with rapid breathing, tachycardia, sweating, and increased muscle tone. Such a person looks awake but typically is unresponsive to environmental stimuli and, if awakened, is disoriented and confused. The typical duration is usually short (seconds to minutes), followed by a return to sleep. There is usually amnesia for the episode after awakening.[14,18,25] Attacks represent partial arousals from deep sleep and may be triggered by sleep-disruptive phenomena such as untreated sleep apnea syndrome, periodic limb movements, pain, and environmental noise. As with other disorders of arousal, there is a strong genetic component, and individuals commonly report a family history of sleep terrors and other disorders of arousal. The prevalence of sleep terrors has been reported between 1% and 7% in children and in 2% of adults.[26] Although night terror episodes are not strongly associated with violence to others, there is a risk when the individual is confronted or brought out of the condition.

Sleepwalking (Somnambulism)

Sleepwalking consists of a series of complex behaviors that are initiated during slow-wave sleep and results in walking or other behaviors during sleep.[14] Typically, the individual sits up in bed during the first third of the night, looks around with a blank stare, and exhibits some repetitive motor automatisms, such as picking at clothes or linens. The somnambulist typically moves about with eyes open and may be able to navigate with some difficulty in familiar settings. The somnambulist lacks the ability to recognize faces or identify family members or friends who may be trying to prevent injury. The somnambulist may walk around the bedroom, enter other rooms, or even leave the house. During the episodes, which usually last 15 minutes or less, there is decreased awareness and impaired responsiveness to surroundings; the individual is difficult to arouse. Accordingly, there is a clinical picture of clumsiness, lack of coordination, and accident proneness—for example, tripping over furniture, sustaining cuts after walking into mirrors, falling down stairs, and even walking through a window. Complex behaviors such as cooking, eating, or driving may occur. Sleepwalking episodes usually terminate by the patient's returning to bed and resuming sleep. Sleepwalkers may also awaken to find themselves in inappropriate places (e.g., in the neighbor's yard or outside in freezing weather without proper clothing). Up to 40% of children experienced at least one sleepwalking episode during childhood, and 2% to 3% of children sleepwalk more than once per month. Between 2% and 3% of adults in the general population sleepwalk.[26,27]

Attempts to awaken a sleepwalker usually fail to produce arousal and may lead to aggressive and violent responses.[14,18,25] Sleepwalkers do not seek out their victims; rather, the victims of sleepwalking violence typically seek out the sleepwalker and accidentally provoke violent defensive behaviors. Cases of sleepwalking violence, including homicidal somnambulism, have been described in the literature and often appear in the news.[28–30]

REM-SLEEP PARASOMNIAS

REM-associated parasomnias include nightmares, REM-sleep behavior disorder, and hypnagogic and hypnopompic hallucinations. One of the cardinal features of REM sleep is the active inhibition of skeletal muscle activity. Skeletal muscle atonia during REM sleep occurs in the context of a highly active brain and prevents sleepers from acting out their dreams.

REM-Sleep Behavior Disorder

REM-sleep behavior disorder is the best-studied REM-sleep parasomnia. The prevalence of violent behavior associated with REM-sleep behavior disorder is 0.5% in the general population.[17] Unlike NREM parasomnias, REM-sleep behavior disorder is more common in the elderly. The age of onset is typically between 50 and 60. Men are affected more than women, and in many individuals there may be a subclinical prodrome that can last for decades. The pathophysiology of REM-sleep behavior disorder is believed to relate to dysfunction of the skeletal muscle atonia that normally accompanies REM sleep, leading to dream enactment. REM-sleep behavior disorder occurs while the patient is fully asleep, and its related behaviors are not due to partial arousals. It is most often considered a prodromal symptom of or secondary to a variety of severe neurodegenerative disorders such as parkinsonism and multiple system atrophy. In a recent case series, 30% to 50% of patients initially presenting with symptoms of REM-sleep behavior disorder went on to develop a neurodegenerative disorder within 10 years.[31]

In a series of cases, violence was associated with the acting out of manifest dream content.[32] In REM-sleep behavior disorder the sleeper's enacted dreams are more affectively laden and may have threatening or violent content of the person being pursued, in danger, or fighting. Upon awakening, such persons relate emotions of fear and are able to recall vivid dreams, usually of a threatening nature. Behaviors reported in individuals with REM-sleep behavior disorder include limb and body jerking, punching, kicking, shouting, swearing, leaping from bed, running into walls or furniture, and striking and choking the bed partner. Since episodes occur during REM sleep, behaviors may recur in a cyclical fashion, every 90 minutes or so throughout the course of sleep. The frequency of dream enactment ranges from a few times a week to nightly.

REM-sleep-related behaviors may result in very serious injuries to patients or their bed partners. Reported injuries include lacerations, fractures, falls, and even subdural hematomas.[33] While patients typically present for medical attention complaining of injurious behaviors toward themselves or their bed partners, violence is usually not concordant with the patient's character.[28,33] This fact is important when expert witnesses are asked to look for the presence or absence of criminal intent. In the case of a potential REM-sleep behavior disorder diagnosis, a sleep laboratory evaluation may be of use in that deficits in the control of voluntary muscle activity are chronic and considered a biologic marker of this disorder.

SEXUAL BEHAVIOR DURING SLEEP

Sexual behavior during sleep is a controversial topic in sleep medicine but one that has found its way into court. The term *sleep behavior during sex* has been used interchangeably with *sleepsex* and *sexsomnia*. Some scientists suggest the term *abnormal sexual behavior during sleep* to distinguish this disorder from common, normal sexual occurrences during sleep, such as nocturnal erection (nocturnal penile tumescence) and vaginal lubrication. Regardless of the terminology, the phenomenon is recognized as a NREM parasomnia variant of confusional arousal,[34–36] but without a unique diagnosis either in the *ICSD-3*[13] or in the *DSM-5*.[12] The prevalence is unknown in the general population, but researchers speculate that it is more common than reported in the literature.[12,37] For forensic purposes, sexsomnia has been considered a variant of sleepwalking.[38]

Exploring the etiology of sexual behavior during sleep, Schenck and colleagues developed a classification of sleep-related disorders and abnormal sexual behaviors during sleep.[39] Based on this schema, sexual behavior during sleep can arise in different categories, parasomnias being only one of them. Other categories include sleep-related sexual seizures, sleep disorders with abnormal sexual behaviors during wakefulness and wake–sleep transitions (as seen in Klein-Levin syndrome), severe chronic insomnia, and restless leg syndrome.[39] Sexual behavior in sleep most often occurs between consenting adults with established sexual relationships in their usual sleeping location. Much more rarely, an individual may arise in a sleepwalking state, walk to another area of the house, and get into bed with someone other than his or her regular partner.

Various acts have been observed and/or reported with sexual behavior during sleep, ranging from sexual sounds to violent sexual events. Authors typically have classified these occurrences based on either the overt behavior or the behavior's effect on the bed partner. Only a single episode of sexual behavior in sleep—masturbation in a female patient—has ever been documented in the sleep laboratory.[40] It occurred following an arousal from deep sleep, lending support to the theory that sexual behavior during sleep is a variant of confusional arousal.

Regardless of the act, it is speculated that many of these cases go unreported and therefore untreated because of embarrassment surrounding these activities.[37,41] Among those patients with sexual behavior during sleep, it is estimated to take 10 to 15 years before it is brought to medical attention.[37] This is concerning, as these persons pose a danger to themselves and/or others.[37] Often, as a result, researchers see only those extreme cases involving sexual assault.

PARASOMNIAS AND THE EXPERT WITNESS

Criminal cases involving parasomnias can be especially contentious because of the difficulty attributing sleep states to an individual retrospectively, the variable interpretation of behavior, and the ever-present question of malingering. Expert witnesses will be called on to explain the causal nexus between parasomnias and behavior and to interpret sleep laboratory findings. Since the scientific study of sleep cuts across disciplines, courts may require testimony from various sleep medicine experts in areas such as sleep behavior and sleep physiology.

To establish that an individual is culpable of a crime, the prosecution must prove the presence of *actus reus* and *mens rea* at the time of the crime. The *actus reus* element represents the culpable act involved in a crime, while the *mens rea* element represents the guilty intent to commit a crime. Invalidation of either element by the defense will eliminate or reduce criminal culpability. In cases of alleged sleepwalking during a crime, it is the *actus reus* requirement that is most often targeted; this is because *actus reus* requires that the alleged guilty act is voluntary. The Model Penal Code (MPC) states that "a person is not guilty of an offense unless his liability is based on conduct that includes a voluntary act or the omission to perform an act of which he is physically capable."[42] Further, the MPC specifically states that bodily movements during unconsciousness or sleep are not considered voluntary acts.[42] The rationale is that a sleeping person is not able to consider the consequences of behavior or to refrain from behavior. Grant points out that, theoretically, sleepwalking defenses may be viewed as negating either the *mens rea* or the *actus reus* requirements, eliminating criminal culpability either because of the absence of the required mental state (guilty intent) or because the defendant did not act voluntarily.[43] Accordingly, expert testimony will address whether a parasomnia deprived the defendant of one of these elements.

LEGAL DEFENSES IN PARASOMNIA CASES

Historically, the sleepwalking defense has involved the legal theories of automatism, unconsciousness, and insanity.[44] While outside of the United States the sleepwalking defense has generally used the automatism defense, U.S. courts have used all three defenses. Automatism is described as automatic, unconscious, and involuntary behaviors in which a person is capable of action but is not conscious of it.[45] Accordingly, the automatism defense negates the *actus reus* requirement of a *voluntary* act.

In the United Kingdom, Australia, and Canada, the legal defense of automatism has been explicitly divided into two categories, insane and noninsane automatism.[46] The Canadian case *R. v. Quick* discussed this distinction—*noninsane automatism* being caused by external factors, such as hypoglycemia due to injected insulin, and *insane automatism* being caused by internal factors, such as organic disorders or mental illness.[47] This distinction is important when considering the consequences of acquittal associated with each defense. An acquittal based on an *insane* automatism defense would result in commitment to a mental institution; a successful *noninsane* automatism defense results in a complete release from custody. Canadian law may also recognize a type of automatism akin to insanity but brought about by severe alcohol intoxication.[48,49]

Despite this legal distinction and the growth of scientific knowledge regarding parasomnias, the sleepwalking defense was once categorized as a noninsane automatism defense in the UK and Canada.[50] Eventually, the UK and Canada abandoned that view of the defense. In the UK, the change in the view of sleepwalking as a noninsane automatism to insane automatism occurred in the 1991 case *R. v. Burgess*.[51] This change was based on an analysis of whether sleepwalking occurred secondary to internal or external factors and the proposition that disorders resulting from internal factors are more likely to recur and put the public at risk. Nevertheless, a finding of insane automatism only occasionally resulted in a hospital order, and some judges simply acquitted defendants when juries found they had been in a state of sleepwalking-related automatism.[52] More recently, the UK approach has grown even more confusing as some judges have required defendants claiming sleepwalking—legally an insane automatism—to be evaluated according to Section 12 of the Mental Health Act of 1983.[53] Thus, some defendants presenting sleepwalking defenses were sent to be evaluated not by sleep experts but by psychiatrists trained to evaluate severe mental disorders such as schizophrenia.[54]

In Canada, sleepwalking had been considered a noninsane automatism, as demonstrated in *R. v. Parks*.[55] In 1987, Parks was accused of killing his mother-in-law and seriously injuring his father-in-law with a knife after driving 18 km from his home to theirs. He was acquitted of all charges. More recently, in the prosecution's appeal of *Luedecke*, the Ontario Supreme Court ruled that sleepwalking was to be considered an insane automatism. This was premised on the view that Luedecke and others with similar findings continued to present a danger to the public.[56]

The sleepwalking defense in the United States has rarely been asserted; as a result, American courts have been inconsistent in their response to it.[57] In these cases, American courts have variably applied the automatism, unconsciousness, and insanity defenses. The first successful sleepwalking defense case in the United States occurred in Massachusetts in 1846.[58] In that case, Albert Tirrell was accused of murdering a prostitute and setting fire to a brothel. There was medical testimony that the victim's wounds could have been self-inflicted.[59] Dr. Samuel Woodward of Worcester testified that Tirrell should be acquitted because he was asleep and did not know what he was doing.[60] The jury instructions directed that a finding of somnambulism would be equivalent to insanity, resulting in acquittal. Tirrell was acquitted after two hours of jury deliberation.

Subsequent to *Tirrell*, American courts used varied approaches to the sleepwalking defense. In the 1879 decision in *Fain v. Commonwealth*, the Court of Appeals of Kentucky found that a defendant was unconscious when he shot and killed his victim during sleep and accordingly was unable to understand the consequences of his behavior.[61] The sleepwalking defense was also viewed as subsumed within the "unconsciousness defense" in a 1974 California case, *People v. Sedeno*.[62] U.S. courts have also permitted the automatism defense in sleepwalking cases. In the 1997 decision in *McClain v. Indiana*, the Supreme Court of Indiana held that a criminal defendant was entitled to present evidence of sleepwalking behaviors as an automatism defense, which highlighted the absence of a necessary component of the *actus reus*—the culpable act.[63] Despite the use of the automatism defense and the unconsciousness defense in various American jurisdictions, Horn notes that their distinction has diminished, and both are functionally equivalent.[57] In fact, many American courts use the terms *automatism defense* and *unconsciousness defense* synonymously.[64]

Are Sleepwalkers Insane?

The sleepwalking defense has also been considered a variant of the insanity defense in the United States. The insanity defense undermines the *mens rea* requirement by establishing that at the time of the crime, a mental disease or defect was present that impaired the defendant's ability to know or appreciate the nature of his act or to conform his behavior to the requirements of the law. In *Tibbs v. Commonwealth* (1910), the Court of Appeals of Kentucky held that the only defense available for acts occurring during sleepwalking was the insanity defense.[65] In *Bradley v. State* (1925), the Court of Criminal Appeals of Texas overturned a murder conviction, holding that the trial court erred in not applying the insanity defense where the defendant claimed to be sleepwalking at the time of the crime.[66]

Later cases clearly opposed the use of the insanity defense in sleepwalking cases. In *State v. Caddell*, the Supreme Court of North Carolina, while acknowledging sleepwalking as a form of unconsciousness, stated that the defenses of insanity and unconsciousness are distinct because "unconsciousness at the time of the alleged criminal act need not be the result of a disease or defect of the mind" (p. 360).[64] The Supreme Court of Wyoming also made this distinction in *Fulcher v. State* (1981).[67] The Wyoming court reasoned that without such distinction a person who was unconscious but not mentally ill at the time of the crime would face commitment at a mental institution upon acquittal. The court stated that commitment of such an individual to a mental institution for rehabilitation would be of no value. The Supreme Court of Indiana, citing *Fulcher*, in *McClain v. Indiana* agreed with this distinction and held that the automatism defense was more appropriate than the insanity defense in sleepwalking cases.

Sexual Behavior During Sleep and Automatism

Criminal cases implicating sexual behavior during sleep have caused a medicolegal conundrum. In Canadian jurisprudence this behavior falls under automatism, described as "the state of a person who, though capable of action, is not conscious of what he is doing…in other words, an unconscious involuntary action."[68] The controversial nature of these cases is illustrated by the 2008 acquittal of Jan Luedecke in Ontario. Luedecke, a landscaper with a history of somnambulism as a child and adult, attended a party at which he drank alcohol to intoxication and fell asleep next to a woman, who later accused him of rape. During the trial, he presented a noninsane automatism defense based on his claim that he suffered from sexsomnia. The court accepted Luedecke's defense based on a multitude of factors, including his history of somnambulism, precipitating factors (alcohol consumption and sleep deprivation), his polysomnogram test results, the fact that his was his first criminal offense, and his cooperation with officials at the time of the event. To the court's discredit, the extent to which drugs and alcohol played a role in his behavior was one of the factors that led to his acquittal. The defense's argument that the excessive consumption of alcohol can induce somnambulism is a controversial claim.[69] Also, the court was aware that Luedecke was wearing a condom during the incident, which could have served as an indicator of conscious awareness of his actions and the potential consequences of unprotected sex. Worse, there was no rebuttal expert testimony from the Crown; the court rejected the Crown's proposed expert on the basis of qualifications. In a subsequent Canadian case, the sexsomnia defense was rejected after a defense expert provided unscientific opinions regarding the relationship between alcohol and sleepwalking and credible rebuttal expert testimony was presented by the Crown.[70,71] Following the expert testimony in that case, the defendant abandoned his sexsomnia claim and then argued that the sex was consensual.

In the United States, several cases have involved the sexsomnia defense, although the judgments rarely favor the defense. In 2001, Adam Kieczykowski was charged with entering dormitory rooms at the University of Massachusetts without permission and inappropriately touching a woman.[72] He had a significant personal and family history of sleepwalking and had no recollection of the events. In addition to his defense claims, several of the victims were unable to identify Kieczykowski as the attacker, resulting in his acquittal.[73] In 2005, Richard Anderson of Chelmsford, Massachusetts, was accused of sexually molesting two adolescent girls on two different occasions.[74] At the grand jury hearing one of the girls testified that he had to be sleeping during the event because he was snoring. Anderson pled guilty to lesser charges of assault and battery and served 3 years' probation, which included court-ordered sex-offender counseling. Here, *unconsciousness* negated the more severe charges and permitted plea negotiation.

Does a Legal Trend Exist?

There are too few judicial opinions to generate firm inferences as to how judges and juries integrate sleep science into deliberations on moral matters. Thus, while the science may be improving, other factors, such as public sentiment and lawyering skills, remain in the calculus of who gets acquitted. Most criminal defendants settle by way of plea negotiations, leaving a dearth of cases to analyze. Sleep-related behavior is so rarely employed in defense of criminal charges that it is premature to attempt a trend analysis; parasomnia is not necessarily the defense *du jour*. Defendants who are acquitted at trial for murder do not have appeal decisions. The remaining cases show no overall pattern.

Martin has collected several modern examples, beginning with the 1981 trial of Steven Steinberg in Arizona.[30] Steinberg stabbed his wife to death, denied any memory of it, and claimed that he was sleepwalking. His expert psychiatrist called it a dissociative reaction and the jury found Steinberg temporarily insane—a complete defense. Arizona had tightened its law of insanity by the time Scott Falater went on trial in 1999; he had stabbed his wife to death in 1997. Also claiming sleepwalking, his behavior after the incident behavior was too complex and goal-directed to convince a jury he was actually asleep.[75] He used the services of the sleep expert who had examined the Canadian defendant Parks. The prosecution's testimony focused on the degree of cognitive ability required for Falater's behavior.[76] The jury could not accept the complexity of the behavior as sleep-related, causing the defense's testimony to appear contrived. Similar failed defenses were seen in Pennsylvania and California.[29] Defendant Ricksgers, in a 1994 Pennsylvania case, claimed his wife killing was brought on by sleep apnea. Defendant Reitz, in a 2001 California case, claimed that he had been a lifelong sleepwalker. Reitz's sleepwalking defense was foiled by his history of violence against his lover.

FORENSIC ASSESSMENTS IN PARASOMNIA-RELATED CASES

The diagnostic evaluation for a sleepwalking defense is primarily based on the clinical history and a detailed description of behaviors immediately before, during, and after the criminal act. Box 7.2 includes recommended clinical guidelines for the assessment of sleep-related violence claims. Sleep laboratory evaluations have not been shown to be of value in the evaluation of sleepwalking as a defense for criminal acts. Published research has shown there are no reliable biologic markers for sleepwalking that can be identified in a sleep study. Although studies have shown that patients with NREM parasomnias tend to have more sleep fragmentation in slow-wave sleep, the causal relationship between the two has yet be elucidated.[77,78] Even patients with a history of frequent NREM parasomnias are very unlikely to have an episode in the sleep laboratory. The use of provocative tests after the fact has been suggested, but this test lacks validation or normative data.

Also, the aim of the criminal defense should be to prove that the defendant was in a sleepwalking state at the time of the crime, not that there may be signs of sleepwalking 6 months or later when the sleep studies are conducted. However, potential triggers of sleepwalking such as snores, apneas, and leg movements may be identified during sleep studies—although the incidence of these symptoms is significantly greater than that of sleepwalking and the overwhelming majority of patients with these symptoms do not present with sleepwalking. Alcohol, although an inducer of sleep, has been shown to prolong NREM sleep and decrease REM sleep during the first half of the night.[69,79] In chronic drinkers these effects can last years after sobriety.[80]

Box 7.2: CLINICAL GUIDELINES FOR ASSESSING POSSIBLE
SLEEP-RELATED VIOLENT BEHAVIOR

1. There should be a reason by history to suspect a bona fide sleep disorder. Similar episodes, with benign or morbid outcome, should have occurred previously.
2. The duration of action is usually brief, although longer episodes may occur.
3. The action is usually abrupt, immediate, impulsive and senseless—without apparent motivation.
4. The behavior, although ostensibly purposeful, is completely inappropriate for the total situation.
5. The behavior is out of waking character for the individual.
6. There is no evidence of premeditation.
7. The victim is someone who happened to be in close proximity.
8. The victim is someone who encountered, touched or blocked the sleepwalker's behavior.
9. The victim's own behavior may have provoked the sleepwalker's response.
10. Sleepwalkers do not seek out victims.
11. There should be no evidence of conscious awareness.
12. There should be no evidence of higher cognitive functioning— memory from before the episode, formation of memory during the episode, planning, intent, or social interaction.
13. Sleepwalkers generally have complete amnesia for the episode.
14. Occasionally, sleepwalkers may have a memory of a brief, static dreamlike image that occurred during the episode, but no memory of their actual behaviors.
15. After regaining consciousness, there is often bewilderment over what occurred and their role in it.
16. After regaining consciousness, there is no attempt to conceal evidence of their behaviors.
17. Behaviors do not occur directly from wakefulness.
18. Behaviors most often occur from deep sleep—1–3 hours after sleep onset.
19. Behaviors are often preceded by sleep deprivation and situational stress.
20. Often behaviors are associated with a trigger that causes arousal from sleep such as sleep-disordered breathing, leg movements, sounds, or touch.
21. Behaviors are not associated with alcohol or alcohol intoxication.

22. Polysomnography (sleep studies) performed months or years after the index episode cannot determine if the individual was in a sleep-walking state at the time of the incident.

Adapted from Cramer-Bornemann MA, Mahowald MW. Sleep forensics. In: Kryger MH, Roth T, Dement WC, eds. Principles and Practice of Sleep Medicine, *5th ed. St. Louis, MO: Elsevier Saunders; 2011: 725–737.*

The workup for disorders of arousal includes a psychiatric history (including family and personal history of sleep disorders and collateral history from the bed partner) and complete physical and neurologic examinations.[36] Although a full-night polysomnogram with audiovisual monitoring is warranted, it may not capture these episodes. For the purposes of a forensic evaluation of a disorder of arousal, the "history must include: 1) detailed description of the event and characterization of the degree of amnesia; 2) current, past, and family sleep disorders; 3) social habits, such as sleep deprivation, drug use, and alcohol intake; 4) current and past medical records and family medical history; 5) employment records (to check for difficulties related to sleep disorders); 6) determination of the frequency of abnormal behavior and its stereotypic nature. Furthermore, the history must include interviews with the spouse or bed partner and family members, questioning the following items: description of the event and prior ones; timing of the behavior; age of onset and associated life events or trauma; degree of amnesia noted; attitude after previous sleep-related disturbances" (p. 335).[41]

CONCLUSION

As we learn more about the pathophysiology of the parasomnias, clinicians and expert witnesses alike will benefit from understanding the boundaries of consciousness and sleep states. At present, science has much to offer criminal justice, as long as we are modest in our claims and evaluate all cases thoroughly and objectively. Knowing about the range of REM and NREM disorders and their presentations will enable forensic professionals to distinguish legitimate from malingered cases. However, criminal matters require accurate, reliable, relevant, honest, and helpful expert testimony. Care must be taken not to prejudice jurors with scientific findings of dubious quality. Since all postarrest polysomnographic studies reflect only present tendencies, if anything, expert witnesses must be especially circumspect in drawing any inferences about a state of consciousness during the commission of a crime.

The problem for the forensic professional is "connecting the dots" between laboratory findings and an individual criminal defendant. Although we endorse the use of polysomnographic studies, all parties must appreciate that, like EEGs, they may or may not display the physiology in question. Perhaps expert witnesses can benefit from the type of logic employed by prosecutors and many jurors—that documented behaviors before, during, and after a criminal act are most indicative of degree of awareness. The commonsense criteria for authenticity articulated by Ray[5] and Bonkalo[3] remain intuitively sound and will therefore carry the most probative weight.

REFERENCES

1. Shakespeare W. *Macbeth*. Act V, Scene 1, Lines 10–12.
2. Plante DT, Winkelman JW. Parasomnias: psychiatric considerations. *Sleep Med Clin.* 2008; 3: 217–229.
3. Bonkalo A. Impulsive acts and confusion will states during incomplete arousal from sleep: criminological and forensic implications. *Psychiatric Q.* 1974; 48: 400–409.
4. Rush B. Of dreaming, incubus, or night mare, and somnambulism. In: Rush B. *Medical Inquiries and Observations upon the Diseases of the Mind*, 5th ed. Philadelphia, PA: Grigg and Elliot; 1835: 298–303.
5. Ray I. *A Treatise on the Medical Jurisprudence of Insanity*, 3rd ed. Boston, MA: Little, Brown, and Company; 1853.
6. American Academy of Sleep Medicine. *International Classification of Sleep Disorders*. Westchester, IL: American Academy of Sleep Medicine; 2005.
7. American Psychiatric Association. *Diagnostic and Statistical Manual of Mental Disorders*, 2nd ed. Washington, DC: American Psychiatric Association; 1968.
8. American Psychiatric Association. *Diagnostic and Statistical Manual of Mental Disorders*, 3rd ed. Washington, DC: American Psychiatric Association; 1980.
9. American Psychiatric Association. *Diagnostic and Statistical Manual of Mental Disorders*, 3rd ed.—Revised. Washington, DC: American Psychiatric Association; 1987.
10. American Psychiatric Association. *Diagnostic and Statistical Manual of Mental Disorders*, 4th ed. Washington, DC: American Psychiatric Association; 1994.
11. American Psychiatric Association. *Diagnostic and Statistical Manual of Mental Disorders*, 4th ed.—Text Revision. Washington, DC: American Psychiatric Association; 2000.
12. American Psychiatric Association. *Diagnostic and Statistical Manual of Mental Disorders*, 5th ed. Washington, DC: American Psychiatric Association; 2013.
13. American Academy of Sleep Medicine. *International Classification of Sleep Disorders*, 3rd ed. Westchester, IL: American Academy of Sleep Medicine; 2014.
14. American Academy of Sleep Medicine. *International Classification of Sleep Disorders*. Westchester, IL: American Academy of Sleep Medicine; 2005.
15. Carskadon MA, Dement WC. Normal human sleep: an overview. In: Kryger MH, Roth T, Dement WC, eds. *Principles and Practice of Sleep Medicine*. Philadelphia, PA: Elsevier Saunders; 2005: 13–23.

16. Broughton RJ. NREM arousal parasomnias. In: Kryger MH, Roth T, Dement WC, eds. *Principles and Practice of Sleep Medicine*. Philadelphia, PA: W.B. Saunders Company; 2000: 693–706.

17. Ohayon MM, Caulet M, Priest RG. Violent behavior during sleep. *J Clin Psychiatry*. 1997; 58: 369–376.

18. Winkelman JW, Herzog DB, Fava, M. The prevalence of sleep-related eating disorder in psychiatric and non-psychiatric populations. *Psychol Med*. 1999; 29: 1461–1466.

19. Bassetti C, Vella S, Donati F, Wielepp P, Weder B. SPECT during sleepwalking. *Lancet*. 2000; 356: 484–485.

20. Mason T, Pack A. Sleep terrors in childhood. *J Pediatr*. 2005; 147: 388–392.

21. Capp PK, Pearl PL, Lewin D. Pediatric sleep disorders. *Primary Care*. 2005; 32: 549–562.

22. Kotagal S, Pianosi P. Sleep disorders in children and adolescents. *Br Med J*. 2006; 332: 828–832.

23. Mason T, Pack A. Pediatric parasomnias. *Sleep*. 2007; 30: 141–151.

24. Petit D, Touchette E, Tremblay RE, Boivin M, Montplasir J. Dysomnias and parasomnias in early childhood. *Pediatrics*. 2007; 119: 1016–1025.

25. Mahowald MW, Cramer-Bornemann MA. NREM sleep-arousal parasomnias. In: Kryger MH, Roth T, Dement WC, eds. *Principles and Practice of Sleep Medicine*. Philadelphia, PA: Elsevier Saunders; 2005: 889–896.

26. Ohayon MM, Guilleminault C, Priest RG. Night terrors, sleepwalking, and confusional arousals in the general population: their frequency and relationship to other sleep and mental disorders. *J Clin Psychiatry*. 1999; 60: 268–276.

27. Klackenberg G. Somnambulism in childhood—prevalence, course and behavioral correlations. A prospective longitudinal study (6–16 years). *Acta Paediatr Scand*. 1982; 71: 495–499.

28. Cartwright R. Sleepwalking violence: a sleep disorder, a legal dilemma, and a psychological challenge. *Am J Psychiatry*. 2004; 161: 1149–1158.

29. Lyon L. 7 criminal cases that invoked the 'sleepwalking defense'. *U.S. News & World Report*. May 8, 2009. Available online at http://health.usnews.com/articles/health/sleep/2009/05/08/7-criminal-cases-that-invoked-the-sleepwalking-defense.html. Accessed November 12, 2013.

30. Martin L. Can sleepwalking be a murder defense? Available online at http://www.lakesidepress.com/pulmonary/Sleep/sleep-murder.htm. Accessed November 12, 2013.

31. Boeve BF, Silber MH, Ferman TJ, et al. Clinicopathologic correlations in 172 cases of rapid eye movement sleep behavior disorder with or without a coexisting neurologic disorder. *Sleep Med*. 2013; 14: 754–762.

32. Hempel AG, Felthous AR, Meloy JR. Psychotic dream-related aggression: a critical review and proposal. *Aggression and Violent Behavior*. 2003; 8: 599–620.

33. Mahowald MW, Schenck CH. REM sleep parasomnias. In: Kryger MH, Roth T, Dement WC, eds. *Principles and Practice of Sleep Medicine*. Philadelphia, PA: Elsevier Saunders; 2005: 897–916.

34. Shapiro C, Federoff J, Trajanovic N. Sexual behaviour in sleep—a newly described parasomnia. *Sleep Res*. 1996; 25: 367.

35. Shapiro C, Trajanovic N, Federoff J. Sexsomnia—a new parasomnia. *Can J Psychiatry*. 2003; 48: 311–317.

36. Zaharna M, Budur K, Noffsinger S. Sexual behavior during sleep: convenient alibi or parasomnia. *Current Psychiatry*. 2008; 7: 21–30.
37. Mangan MA. A phenomenology of problematic sexual behavior occurring in sleep. *Arch Sex Behav*. 2004; 33: 287–293.
38. Rosenfeld D, Elhajjar A. Sleepsex: a variant of sleepwalking. *Arch Sex Behav*. 1998; 27: 269–278.
39. Schenck, CH, Arnulf I, Mahowald MW. Sleep and sex: what can go wrong? A review of the literature on sleep related disorders and abnormal sexual behaviors and experiences. *Sleep*. 2007; 30: 683–702.
40. Cicolin A, Tribolo A, Giordano A, et al. Sexual behaviors during sleep associated with polysomnographically confirmed parasomnia overlap disorder. *Sleep Med*. 2011; 12: 523–528.
41. Guilleminault C, Moscovitch A, Yuen K, Poyares D. Atypical sexual behavior during sleep. *Psychosomatic Med*. 2002; 64: 328–336.
42. American Law Institute. *Model Penal Code*. Philadelphia, PA: American Law Institute; 1962.
43. Grant E. While you were sleeping or addicted: a suggested expansion of the automatism doctrine to include an addiction defense. *University of Illinois Law Review*. 2000; 2000: 997–1023.
44. Bourget D, Whitehurst L. Amnesia and crime. *J Am Acad Psychiatry Law*. 2007; 35: 469–480.
45. Arboleda-Florez J. On automatism. *Curr Opin Psychiatry*. 2002; 15: 569–576.
46. Samuels A, O'Driscoll C, Allnutt S. When killing isn't murder: psychiatric and psychological defences to murder when the insanity defence is not applicable. *Austral Psychiatry*. 2007; 15: 474–479.
47. *R. v. Quick* (1973). QB 910.
48. Bondy SJ. A summary of public consultation on reform of the Criminal Code of Canada as related to a defense of self-induced intoxication resulting in automatism. *Contemporary Drug Problems*. 1996; 23: 583–593.
49. Kalant, H. Intoxicated automatism: legal concept vs. scientific evidence. *Contemporary Drug Problems*. 1996; 23: 631–648.
50. Fenwick P. Somnambulism and the law: a review. *Behavioral Science and the Law*. 1987; 5: 343–347.
51. *R. v. Burgess* (1991). 2 QB 92.
52. *R. v. James Bilton*, United Kingdom, 2005.
53. Mental Health Act, 1983, Section 12 (England).
54. *R. v. Thompson*, Nottingham, UK, 2010.
55. *R. v. Parks* (1992). 2 SCR 871.
56. *R. v. Luedeke* (2008). 2008 ONCA 716.
57. Horn M. A rude awakening: what to do with the sleepwalking defense? *Boston College Law Review*. 2004; 46: 149–182.
58. Brown SG. *The Life of Rufus Choate*, 6th ed. Boston, MA: Little, Brown, and Co.; 1898.
59. Hill CH. Memoir of the Hon. Rufus Choate. *Proceedings of the Massachusetts Historical Society*. 1896; 11: 124–155.
60. J.M.S. The trial of Albert John Tirrell. *Prisoner's Friend*. April 1, 1846: 50.
61. *Fain v. Commonwealth*, 78 Ky. 183 (1879).
62. *People v. Sedeno*, 518 P.2d 913 (Cal. 1974).
63. *McClain v. Indiana*, 678 N.E.2d 104 (Ind. 1997).
64. *State v. Caddell*, 215 S.E.2d 348 (NC 1975).

65. *Tibbs* v. *Commonwealth*, 128 S.W. 871 (Ky. 1910).
66. *Bradley* v. *State*, 277 S.W. 147 (Tex. Crim. App. 1925).
67. *Fulcher* v. *State*, 633 P.2d 142 (Wy. 1981).
68. Buchanan A. Sleepwalking and indecent exposure. *Medicine, Science and the Law.* 1991; 31: 38–40.
69. Pressman MR, Mahowald MW, Schenck CH, Cramer-Bornemann MA. Alcohol-induced sleepwalking or confusional arousal as a defense to criminal behavior: a review of scientific evidence, methods and forensic considerations. *J Sleep Res.* 2007; 16: 198–212.
70. Makin K. Judge rejects 'sexsomnia' defence. *The Globe and Mail (Toronto).* May 2, 2009.
71. *R.* v. *Teepell* (2009). Walkerton 05-543.
72. Morgan R. Are you raping your wife in your sleep? *Details.* April 2006. Available online at http://www.details.com/sex-relationships/marriage-and-kids/200604/are-you-raping-your-wife-in-your-sleep. Accessed November 14, 2013.
73. Lindsay J. Man charged with child molestations. *The Milford* (Massachusetts) *Daily News*, March 26, 2005. Available online at http://www.milforddailynews.com/archive/x1612084296. Accessed July 1, 2011.
74. Schenck CH. *Sleep: The Mysteries, the Problems, and the Solutions.* New York: Avery; 2007.
75. Rubin, P. The big sleep. *Phoenix New Times.* February 14, 2002. Available online at http://www.phoenixnewtimes.com/2002-02-14/news/the-big-sleep/. Accessed November 14, 2013.
76. Pressman MR. Response to Rosalind Cartwright's letter to the editor. *Sleep Med Rev.* 2007; 11: 329–333.
77. Espa F, Ondze B, Deglise P, Billiard M, Besset A. Sleep architecture, slow wave activity, and sleep spindles in adult patients with sleepwalking and sleep terrors. *Clin Neurophysiol.* 2000; 111: 929–939.
78. Andersen M, Poyares D, Alves R, Skomro R, Tufik S. Sexsomnia: abnormal sexual behavior during sleep. *Brain Res Rev.* 2007; 56: 271–282.
79. Doghramji K. The effects of alcohol on sleep. *Medscape Family Medicine.* January 27, 2005. Available online at http://www.medscape.org/viewarticle/497982. Accessed November 14, 2013.
80. Brower KJ, Aldrich MS, Hall JM. Polysomnographic and subjective sleep predictors of alcoholic relapse. *Alcoholism Clin Exp Res.* 1998; 22: 1864–1871.

CHAPTER 8

Neuroimaging and Criminal Culpability

SUSAN E. RUSHING AND DANIEL D. LANGLEBEN*

Medical imaging can assist an expert in evaluating the brain structure and function of a forensic examinee. While progress has been made in the research correlating brain functional and structural abnormalities with behavior, the criminal justice system has been cautious in introducing scientific testimony that correlates brain structure and function with behaviors relevant to crime, such as violence. Supported by extensive clinical use, neuropsychological testing and structural imaging in the form of computed tomography (CT) and structural magnetic resonance imaging (MRI) have achieved general acceptance in court. However, functional imaging, such as functional MRI (fMRI) and nuclear medicine techniques such as positron emission tomography (PET) and single photon emission computed tomography (SPECT), have faced more admissibility challenges. While functional imaging is becoming an increasingly important tool in assessing brain-based illness and deficits, we surmise that evidentiary challenges are largely related to the phase of trial in which a functional neuroimaging study is offered as evidence. Scholars have feared that the "seeing is believing" phenomenon may unduly influence jurors. Ethicists have worried about the specter of determinism that may attach to those detected to have brain-based lesions, which have been correlated with violent behaviors. Studies of mock juries suggest that neuroimaging plays little to no role in a jury's finding of guilt or innocence in homicide trials. Whether these data have affected the rate at which functional neuroimaging evidence is currently sought in the guilt phase is unknown. The most prevalent use of neuroimaging in criminal

* Portions of this chapter were previously published as: Rushing SE, Langleben D. Relevant Function: Nuclear Brain Imaging in U.S. Courts. *J Psychiatry Law.* 2011; 39: 567–593. Used with permission from Federal Legal Publications, Inc., Somers, NY.

justice is in the penalty phase of capital trials, where the Supreme Court has relaxed admissibility standards to allow defendants to introduce any evidence that could lead to a sentence less than death. This chapter will focus on the nuclear imaging modalities and include a review of the principles of PET and SPECT and discuss cases where the admissibility of these techniques has been challenged and whether and how nuclear brain imaging can influence the outcome of a criminal trial. The science behind the forensic use of another form of functional imaging, fMRI, is discussed in Chapter 6.

INTRODUCTION TO NUCLEAR MEDICINE IMAGING

PET and SPECT are nuclear medicine techniques that use energy emitted by the decay of radioactive tracers attached to biologically active compounds to produce three-dimensional images reflecting the distribution of these compounds in the internal organs, including the brain. Since SPECT and PET can be sensitive to changes on the order of seconds to minutes, they are considered "functional" imaging techniques. Glucose labeled with fluorine-18 (2-deoxy-2-[^{18}F]-fluoro-D-glucose [FDG]) is the radiopharmaceutical most commonly used in clinical brain PET. ^{18}FDG is taken up by brain cells in the same way as unlabeled glucose, but rather than being metabolized, it becomes trapped in the brain cell. Energy emitted by the decay of ^{18}F, an unstable isotope of fluorine, reflects the amount of radiolabeled glucose taken up by the brain.

Other elements, such as oxygen and nitrogen, can be radiolabeled and their metabolism imaged. FDG-PET is a universally accepted clinical test in the diagnosis and follow-up of malignancy,[1,2] myocardial viability, epilepsy,[3,4] and degenerative brain disease.[5-9] Other relatively common clinical uses include presurgical planning, poststroke evaluation,[10] and evaluation of moderate to severe traumatic brain injury.[11,12] PET is commonly used by forensic medicine practitioners to demonstrate diffuse axonal injury, which is characteristic of mild traumatic brain injury.[13,14] The most common clinical uses of brain SPECT are to characterize neurodegenerative disorders such as dementia, as well as perfusion abnormalities associated with stroke, seizures, inflammation, and trauma.[15] The radioisotope most commonly used in brain SPECT is technetium-99m (^{99m}Tc).[16] Forensic uses of PET and SPECT follow and sometimes jump ahead of the clinical applications of these nuclear medicine techniques. For example, an expert may be asked whether a scan can aid in determining a litigant's state of mind at the time of the crime. In some cases the behavior in question preceded the brain scan by months or even years and any answer will be speculation. Thus, whereas using FDG-PET to support evidence of dementia is relatively straightforward, using it to prove a defendant's inability to control his or her impulses five years prior to the scan is much more controversial. Working knowledge of the basic nuclear medicine techniques and applications is becoming an important skill for forensic psychiatrists.

USE OF NUCLEAR IMAGING IN CRIMINAL TRIALS

For the past decade there has been much debate concerning the admissibility and the appropriateness of expert witnesses discussing brain scans in the courtroom.[17,18] Legal scholars have expressed fears that colorful pictures will distract jurors from the true legal issues they must decide.[19] As this debate has been waged, brain imaging has become an important tool used clinically by physicians to detect potential brain-based explanations for abnormal behavior. While not all abnormal behavior is criminal behavior, some is, and there is the potential for criminal behavior to follow abnormal behavior. We predict that as nuclear imaging and other modes of functional brain imaging such as fMRI enter the realm of standard medical practice, the rate of admission of functional brain scans into evidence will increase dramatically. At present, the phase of trial during which the functional brain scan is offered as evidence is an important variable in whether an admissibility challenge will be raised. Prior to discussing specific examples of evidentiary challenges, we will review basic information about phases of criminal trials.

Trials are divided into four phases: the pretrial phase, the guilt phase, the sentencing phase, and the postconviction relief (or appeal) phase. Psychiatric testimony can be presented during any phase of trial. Prior to trial on the issue of an individual's guilt, attorneys can bring motions before the court. Common pretrial issues raised in criminal trials include whether a defendant is competent to stand trial, whether a defendant was competent to waive *Miranda* rights, whether a juvenile defendant should be tried in the adult justice system, and whether certain types of scientific evidence or testimony will be permitted at trial. The government and the defense will submit pretrial motions, and these motions will be argued prior to the guilt phase of the criminal trial. We will begin by discussing the legal standards for expert testimony and the introduction of scientific evidence. We will then review cases in which the government opposed the introduction of expert testimony and brain scans in criminal trials.

PRETRIAL CHALLENGES TO THE INTRODUCTION OF SCIENTIFIC EVIDENCE AND EXPERT TESTIMONY

The Federal Rules of Evidence govern the introduction of evidence in civil and criminal proceedings in federal courts. The rules of evidence used in many states have been closely modeled on these provisions. Rule 702 addresses testimony by experts as follows:

> If scientific, technical, or other specialized knowledge will assist the trier of fact to understand the evidence or to determine a fact in issue, a witness qualified as an expert by knowledge, skill, experience, training, or education, may testify thereto in the form of an opinion or otherwise, if (1) the testimony is based upon sufficient facts or data, (2) the testimony is the product of reliable principles and methods, and (3) the witness has applied the principles and methods reliably to the facts of the case.[20]

Rule 702 was amended in 2000 to reflect case law, including *Daubert v. Merrell Dow Pharmaceuticals* (1995),[21] which held that Rule 702 of the Federal Rules of Evidence did not incorporate the *Frye* "general acceptance" test[22] as a basis for assessing the admissibility of scientific expert testimony. Despite this change to the Federal Rules of Evidence, the *Frye* standard is maintained in many states, including Alabama, Arizona, California, Florida, Illinois, Kansas, Maryland, Michigan, Minnesota, New Jersey, New York, Pennsylvania, and Washington. In these jurisdictions, scientific procedures, principles, or techniques that may be discussed by the expert during trial must be "generally accepted" by the relevant scientific community. Questions that may arise during trial in a *Frye* state could include "Would other psychiatrists or nuclear medicine physicians also rely on PET for diagnosing or evaluating this disorder?" The opposing side could then refute "general acceptance" by calling an expert who would testify that many psychiatrists and nuclear medicine physicians would not agree that PET could be used to evaluate the condition in question.

The *Daubert* standard was initially touted as a more lenient standard for admission of scientific evidence, but time has proven it effective at limiting admission of scientific evidence that falls short of its criteria. Prior to trial, the judge will review the submitted evidence and determine whether the scientific method or reasoning is valid and could be properly applied to the facts at issue in the case. The judge must consider whether the theory or technique in question can be and has been tested; whether it has been subjected to peer review and publication; its known or potential error rate and the existence and maintenance of standards controlling its operation; and whether it has attracted widespread acceptance within a relevant scientific community. The majority of states' evidentiary standards are based on the *Daubert* standard.

A party that wants to prevent the introduction of scientific evidence to the jury will file a "motion in limine" before trial begins to attempt to exclude presentation of the evidence. Motion in limine will be discussed further in the case examples that follow. In the following section, we will discuss specific case examples in which an evidentiary challenge has arisen to admission of functional brain imaging data. The following case examples were obtained through a search of the medical literature and court documents. No individual discussed below was clinically evaluated by the authors.

PET NOT ADMISSIBLE IN A CASE OF KIDNAPPING BY CESAREAN SECTION

Criminal defendant Lisa Montgomery had an online friendship with her pregnant victim, Bobbie Jo Stinnett. The two had engaged in email exchanges about their respective "pregnancies." Montgomery arranged to meet Stinnett and buy a rat terrier puppy from her. Montgomery strangled the expectant mother, performed a cesarean section, and kidnapped Stinnett's premature baby. Stinnett died but her premature daughter survived. Montgomery crossed state lines with the baby, making her crime a federal offense.

In Montgomery's defense, expert witnesses planned to testify that Montgomery suffered from pseudocyesis, or false pregnancy, a condition that could have led to a diminished capacity finding. Prosecution experts disagreed with the pseudocyesis diagnosis, theorizing that Montgomery was having marital problems and believed a baby would reunite her with her husband. To support the claim of pseudocyesis, a defense expert planned to show that Montgomery had increased activity in her hypothalamus detected on PET. The defense expert would testify that this finding was consistent with the diagnosis of pseudocyesis because the disorder has been hypothesized to be caused by an imbalance in pituitary-ovarian function and dysregulation of the hypothalamus.[23] The government filed a pretrial motion to suppress the discussion of Montgomery's brain scan during her trial for capital murder.

A central question at the evidentiary hearing was whether clinicians generally relied upon PET when diagnosing pseudocyesis. The answer to this question was a prime determinant in whether the scans would be admitted into evidence during the guilt phase of trial. All of the involved experts agreed that neuroimaging confirmation of hypothalamic dysregulation is not part of the clinical workup for pseudocyesis. A second important factor was whether a causal connection could be established between the brain abnormalities demonstrated on PET and the crime that Montgomery committed. The defense expert testified that the abnormalities that appeared in the limbic and somatomotor regions of the brain did not predict behavior and did not cause Montgomery to commit the crime. Therefore, the court concluded that the information that could be displayed in the PET scan would not assist the jury in determining whether Montgomery's brain abnormality caused her criminal behavior. Because PET scans are not used in the diagnostic workup for pseudocyesis and the scan could not assist the trier of fact in determining causation, the scans were excluded from evidence.

PET ADMISSIBLE TO SHOW BRAIN DAMAGE IN A DEFENDANT WITH A BULLET LODGED IN HIS BRAIN

Miguel Carrizalez was charged with two counts of murder, six counts of attempted murder, and gang-related charges in California. He had sustained a gunshot wound to the head and had a bullet lodged in his brain. He claimed incompetence to stand trial due to this severe traumatic brain injury and offered a PET scan in support. The prosecution objected to the admission of the PET scan and an admissibility hearing was held. During the competence hearing, the judge stated that PET studies are "generally accepted in the scientific community and ... are certainly accepted as tools used in clinical settings. And in forensic settings it seems ... there could be testimony as to the areas of the brain that are relevant to the issue of [trial competency]" (pp. 261-262).[24] The PET study was admitted into evidence. The court heard testimony regarding Carrizalez's severe traumatic brain injury and viewed neuroimaging evidence in support of this testimony. Despite this evidence, Carrizalez was found competent to stand trial for capital murder. His trial proceeded and he was convicted of all charges. PET images were presented during the sentencing phase and testimony focused on the severity of his brain injury and subsequent personality changes. The jury did not return a unanimous vote in favor of the death penalty, as required for the imposition of the death penalty in California. The district attorney did not retry the penalty phase, and Carrizalez was sentenced to life without the possibility of parole.

PET ADMISSIBLE TO SUPPORT A CLAIM OF DEMENTIA IN AN ALLEGED MAFIA BOSS

Vincent Gigante, an alleged Mafia boss, was found guilty of a number of federal criminal charges, including conspiracy and racketeering. He was examined by several psychiatrists, who found that he suffered from dementia on clinical examination. His attorneys claimed that he was incompetent to be sentenced due to his dementia. A PET study was submitted in support of this claim. The court admitted the PET evidence but declined to rely upon it. The court noted that the scan was excellent technically but was not conducive to uniform interpretation Specifically, the court was concerned that the controls in the study were not treated with the same psychotropic drugs that Gigante was prescribed, including chlorpromazine, nortryptiline, diazepam, temazepam, and flurazepam. The court noted that if Gigante were taking these medications, they would have a profound effect on the PET metabolic images; however, it was impossible to say what the combined effect would be. Ultimately, Gigante was adjudicated competent and was sentenced to 12 years in federal prison in 1997.

PERSUASIVE IMAGES

Legal and medical scholars alike have feared the effect that images could have on a jury.[25,26] Some scholars fear that a jury will be overly persuaded by alluring images that have been enhanced with bright colors. Further, there is concern that a jury will find images of a misshapen or malfunctioning brain more persuasive than traditional forms of lay or expert testimony.[26]

A study by Gurley and Marcus weighed the effects of structural neuroimaging with MRI when used in support of an insanity defense in a simulated murder trial.[19] In this study, a sample of 400 mock jurors was more likely to find a defendant not guilty by reason of insanity (NGRI) if an MRI showing a brain lesion was presented than if no image was presented. Mock jurors were even more likely to choose NGRI when both expert testimony and neuroimaging were presented than when either type of evidence alone was presented.[19] The results suggested that the combination of expert testimony and imaging can lead jurors to find that a defendant lacked the *mens rea* needed to commit murder.

However, Schweitzer and colleagues failed to find an increase in *mens rea*-specific defenses when brain images were presented to a mock jury.[27] They designed an experiment in which jurors were presented with identical neuroscience expert testimony, with and without the actual brain scan.[27] All jurors heard expert testimony in which the expert stated that the defendant, who was on trial for murder, suffered from a defect in his frontal lobe and that this defect prevented the defendant from premeditating and deliberating about murder. The expert further stated that the defect prevented the defendant from forming the specific intent needed to be guilty of first- or second-degree murder. In one condition, jurors were shown the brain scan demonstrating damage to the frontal lobe. In another condition, jurors were told that a brain scan was conducted and were shown a visual representation in the form of a bar graph demonstrating the defendant's deficit. Another condition included identical testimony but no graphic depiction of the expert's findings. This study tested the hypothesis of whether clear wrongdoing can be neutralized by neuroscience evidence depicting brain malfunction or injury, which supports a *mens rea* (lack of intent) defense.[27] The presence of brain images had no consistent impact on the verdicts or sentences rendered by the mock jurors. Showing brain images to mock jurors also had no impact on jurors' perception of the defendant's criminal responsibility.[27]

In summary, Gurley and Marcus found that brain images could affect mock jurors' findings regarding *mens rea*, whereas Schweitzer's mock jurors were not swayed by the presentation of such images in the guilt phase. Accordingly, the proverbial jury is still out on the actual impact of brain images on jurors. When a defense attorney chooses to display a brain image in the guilt phase of a criminal trial, the image will almost certainly be presented by an expert, who will testify regarding whether the defendant was capable of forming the *mens rea* needed to accomplish the crime. To negate *mens rea*, the expert must believe that a neurologic defect caused the defendant to be unable to form the intent required to constitute a crime. The following case illustrates the limitations a court placed on an expert's discussion of the link between a powerful brain image and a deadly human action.

Herbert Weinstein was a 65-year-old man who strangled his wife to death in their Manhattan apartment and then threw her body out of their 12th-story apartment window. Weinstein's blasé attitude following his arrest caused his defense attorneys to seek a neurologic evaluation of their elderly client with no known history of violence. PET was performed and showed a large arachnoid cyst pressing on the brain and dramatically altering the expected glucose uptake. Since ^{18}FDG PET images reflect the distribution of glucose metabolism, the cyst appeared like a large void in the man's brain because it essentially is a fluid-filled sac that does not metabolize glucose. The prosecution tried to prevent the PET evidence from being admitted at trial, claiming that PET technology was new and not widely accepted.[28] The judge ruled that the defense could show the PET evidence of the arachnoid cyst but would not allow the defense witnesses to tell jurors that arachnoid cysts were associated with violence.[29] Shortly after the ruling on the admissibility hearing, the prosecution offered Weinstein a plea bargain in which he pled guilty to manslaughter, which carried a sentence of 7 to 21 years in prison. Weinstein was offered surgery but never had his cyst removed. He was incarcerated for 12 years and did not engage in any violent acts while in prison. He was granted a conditional release at age 79 and died 2 years after his release.[30]

IMAGES AND *MENS REA*

When nuclear images are admitted into evidence to prove a prima facie element of the crime, namely *mens rea*, admissibility challenges are more likely to arise. Challenges are less likely to prevail if the incomplete defense of diminished capacity or a variant thereof is at issue. When a defendant raises a diminished capacity defense, it is to suggest that he or she was deprived of a normal level of mental wherewithal. Not every state employs this partial defense. In states that do, it can function to reduce the charge of the offense and could be thought of as a non-plea bargain way to receive a discounted sentence. For example, a finding of diminished capacity could reduce a murder charge to manslaughter. In contrast, a finding of insanity is a complete defense to a crime and will result in an NGRI finding.

SPECT was used to support a claim of "diminished actuality" (similar to diminished capacity) in a California murder trial for defendant Peter Chiesa, a 65-year-old retired chemist with multiple medical problems, including vascular dementia, epilepsy, strokes, and a complicated coronary artery bypass surgery.[31] Chiesa called 911 shortly before he walked outside and shot and killed two female neighbors who were clearing wood off a driveway they shared with him. He perceived people to be "stealing" from his property. The defense used SPECT to illustrate that his brain was "misshapen" and "contained holes." The expert witness for the defense witness testified that he was too cognitively disabled to premeditate first-degree murder. The jury did find diminished actuality, convicted him of two counts of second-degree murder, and sentenced him to 80 years in prison.[32] Chiesa applied for "compassionate release" due to an unspecified medical condition in 2012 but his request was denied, in part because he had hit a nurse during his incarceration. The district attorney argued, "He's exercising the same patterns of getting angry about something and lashing out. If he can hit a nurse, he can pull a trigger."[33]

BROADER ADMISSIBILITY OF PET IN SENTENCING

In *Lockett v. Ohio* (1978), the Supreme Court decreed that a defendant facing the death penalty is entitled to present any aspect of character or record and any circumstance of the offense that might serve as a basis for a sentence less than death, regardless of whether the evidence supports a statutorily authorized mitigating factor.[34] In *Tennard v. Dretke* (2004) the Supreme Court stated that any cognitive or neuropsychological impairment may be considered a mitigating factor, even if the impairment bears no direct link with the homicidal behavior.[35] The Supreme Court has afforded constitutional protections for defendants to introduce mitigating evidence in penalty hearings.[36] "[S]tates cannot limit the sentencer's consideration of any relevant circumstances that could cause it to decline to impose the [death] penalty" (p. 281).[37] More particularly, the juror may "not be precluded from considering, as a mitigating factor, any aspect of a defendant's character or record and any of the circumstances of the offense that the defendant proffers as a basis for a sentence less than death" (p. 604).[34]

Evidence of a structural or metabolic brain abnormality could be included as evidence of a severe mental disturbance, a prong that most states and the

federal government include as a mitigating factor in the death penalty statute. Further, most states allow a defendant to present any "other factor" in
the defendant's background, record, or character or any other circumstance
of the offense that might mitigate against imposition of a death sentence.[34]
Functional images of the brain are commonly admitted in death penalty litigation to demonstrate brain abnormalities that a jury could find mitigating.[31]

POSTCONVICTION RELIEF FOLLOWING A DEATH SENTENCE

If an attorney fails to present mitigating evidence, including evidence of
mental illness or extreme emotional distress, a case can be remanded for
ineffective assistance of counsel. The Supreme Court established a two-part
test for ineffective assistance of counsel in *Strickland v. Washington* (1984).[38]
A case may be remanded if a criminal defendant can show that counsel's performance fell below an objective standard of reasonableness and that it gave
rise to a reasonable probability that, if counsel had performed adequately,
the result of the trial or sentencing would have been different.[38]

Defendant Fernando Caro's death sentence was vacated and remanded
for retrial in California because his attorney failed to investigate and present evidence of the impact that exposure to neurotoxicants and child abuse
had on his brain.[39] The court stated that attorneys must cast a wide net for
all relevant mitigating evidence at capital sentencing hearings because "the
Constitution prohibits imposition of the death penalty without adequate
consideration of factors which might evoke mercy" (p. 1227).[39] In detailing
the sort of evidence that should have been considered, the court did not state
that neuroimaging was needed. Rather, it gave an extensive list of circumstances that were likely to lead to brain damage, including that Caro spent
his childhood working and playing in pesticide-soaked fields and that he
bathed in and was fed food cooked in water contaminated with pesticides.
The court noted that Caro worked as a "flagger" for a crop-dusting company
and at a company that made toxic pesticides. He was regularly exposed to
organophosphates, solvents, organochlorines, and carbamates, and he was
poisoned by a number of toxic chemicals at the plant. In addition, he suffered
serious physical abuse and head injuries. Both parents beat him throughout
his childhood, hitting him with closed fists, sticks, belts, work boots, and
tools. Caro also sustained several head injuries as a child: He was born with
a 3-inch lump on his head due to forceps use during his difficult delivery;
a water cooler fell on his head at the age of 3; and he was hit by a car later
that year.[40] If brain damage resulted from these multiple neurologic insults,
the damage could be demonstrated with PET or SPECT. In *Caro*, the court
suggested that it is adequate for counsel to obtain a corroborated injury history listing factors that led to demonstrated cognitive impairment. *Caro* does

not penalize counsel for failing to obtain or present neuroimaging, but other cases have.[41,42]

SPECT has been used as mitigating evidence in criminal trials for capital murder. In *Smith v. Mullin* (2004), the court ordered a resentencing hearing for Smith, a man found guilty and sentenced to death for murdering his wife and her four children from a prior relationship.[41] The court found that the defendant was prejudiced by his counsel's failure to present evidence of his cognitive disabilities and brain damage. The court noted that evidence of his brain damage was shown in SPECT authorized by the court but was not raised by counsel in the original trial.

In Florida, defendant Hoskins challenged the trial court's judgment convicting him of multiple felonies, including first-degree murder, as well as the imposition of the death sentence.[42] Hoskins had an IQ of 71, and an examining physician recommended that PET be ordered as part of the workup for brain damage. The trial court refused to grant the defendant's motion seeking transport to a hospital to have a brain scan performed. This denial limited his defense expert's ability to evaluate the degree of his mental impairment, which is a statutory mitigating factor under Florida law.[43] The appellate court remanded the case, ordering that a brain scan be obtained and consideration of a new penalty phase, in effect overturning Hoskins' death sentence. The decision in this case has led attorneys to seek nuclear medicine studies for many death-eligible defendants in Florida.

Defendant Francis Hernandez's death sentence was vacated because his attorney failed to consult a neurologist, neuropsychologist, or neuropsychiatrist or to arrange for a neurologic examination of the petitioner, despite the fact that he wrote notes in his legal file suggesting that he planned to do so. On appeal the lawyer stated that "evidence of neurological impairment is the type of evidence I wanted because it would have helped to explain and mitigate Francis's state of mind at the time of the killings" (p. 1085).[44]

When an attorney is seeking evidence of brain damage and is considering a nuclear medicine study, it is up to the expert to evaluate the defendant and determine whether there is a sufficient indication for such study. We discourage experts from prescribing nuclear medicine studies or offering interpretations of the results without first evaluating the patient and obtaining appropriate clinical history.

CONCLUSION

Functional brain imaging studies can assist the judge and jury by allowing them to view the inner workings of the defendant's brain. The information yielded through brain scans is not given the same level of relevance in every phase of trial. In some instances, admissibility challenges may arise regarding either the witness' expertise in neuroimaging or the ability of the images to inform the jury about a fact at issue in the trial.

To establish expertise in neuroimaging, the witness must have the appropriate education and training, an adequate and up-to-date knowledge base, and experience using the imaging technique. In addition to familiarity with the anatomy and physiology of the brain regions to be examined, the expert should be prepared to discuss not only the clinical indications and limitations of a specific neuroimaging technique but also such details as the criteria for determination of what constitutes an abnormal finding in a given individual. After it is determined that the expert is qualified to discuss neuroimaging, the court may consider the ability of the brain image to assist the jury in determining a fact at issue in the trial.

Presentation of brain imaging studies during the guilt phase of a criminal trial is more likely to evoke an evidentiary challenge. Evidentiary challenges generally result when a brain imaging study is offered to substantiate a diagnosis, particularly when the imaging study would not generally be used to support such a diagnosis in clinical practice. Evidentiary challenges may also arise when a nuclear imaging study is offered to support a causal link between a brain-based abnormality and violent behavior. Nuclear studies cannot assist the trier of fact in determining whether the defendant committed the act in question. Similarly, brain images cannot help the jury in understanding the mindset of the defendant at the time of the crime, with a few important exceptions. A brain study can demonstrate structural abnormalities such as cysts, tumors, strokes, seizure foci, or tissue atrophy that could lead to functional deficits and as such reduce a defendant's capacity for self-control. Diminished capacity for self-control is not a complete defense to a crime but will decrease criminal culpability and the associated penalty.

As discussed above, the Supreme Court has determined that a defendant's cognitive and neuropsychological limitations must be considered during the sentencing phase in all death penalty cases. Failure to present evidence of intellectual limitations or brain damage has been a factor in overturning death sentences, as evidence of brain-based deficits could assist a jury in understanding the defendant's limitations and could result in a sentence other than death. Neuroimaging studies, such as PET and SPECT, can demonstrate functional abnormalities in brain metabolism and blood flow. As such, brain imaging introduced as mitigating evidence during the sentencing phase of a capital murder trial is unlikely to face an admissibility challenge.

REFERENCES

1. Bomanji JB, Costa DC, Ell PJ. Clinical role of positron emission tomography in oncology. *Lancet Oncol.* 2001; 2(3): 157–164.
2. Necib H, Garcia C, Wagner A, et al. Detection and characterization of tumor changes in ^{18}F-FDG PET patient monitoring using parametric imaging. *J Nucl Med.* 2011; 52(3): 354–361.
3. Kim YK, Lee DS, Lee SK, Chung CK, Chung JK, Lee MC. ^{18}F-FDG PET in localization of frontal lobe epilepsy: comparison of visual and SPM analysis. *J Nucl Med.* 2002; 43(9): 1167–1174.
4. Kim YK, Lee DS, Lee SK, et al. Differential features of metabolic abnormalities between medial and lateral temporal lobe epilepsy: quantitative analysis of ^{18}F-FDG PET using SPM. *J Nucl Med.* 2003; 44(7): 1006–1012.
5. Juh R, Kim J, Moon D, Choe B, Suh T. Different metabolic patterns analysis of parkinsonism on the ^{18}F-FDG PET. *Eur J Radiol.* 2004; 51(3): 223–233.
6. Jeong Y, Cho SS, Park JM, et al. ^{18}F-FDG PET findings in frontotemporal dementia: an SPM analysis of 29 patients. *J Nucl Med.* 2005; 46(2): 233–239.
7. Ishii K, Willoch F, Minoshima S, et al. Statistical brain mapping of ^{18}F-FDG PET in Alzheimer's disease: validation of anatomic standardization for atrophied brains. *J Nucl Med.* 2001; 42(4): 548–557.
8. Desgranges B, Baron JC, Lalevee C, et al. The neural substrates of episodic memory impairment in Alzheimer's disease as revealed by FDG-PET: relationship to degree of deterioration. *Brain.* 2002; 125(Pt 5): 1116–1124.
9. Newberg AB, Alavi A. The role of PET imaging in the management of patients with central nervous system disorders. *Radiol Clin North Am.* 2005; 43: 49–65.
10. Ances BM, Liebeskind DS, Newberg AB, Jacobs DA, Alavi A. Early uncoupling of cerebral blood flow and metabolism after bilateral thalamic infarction. *AJNR Am J Neuroradiol.* 2004; 25(10): 1685–1687.
11. Ruff RM, Crouch JA, Troster AL, et al. Selected cases of poor outcome following minor brain trauma: comparing neuropsychological and positron emission tomography assessment. *Brain Injury.* 1994; 8: 297–308.
12. Bergsneider M, Hovda DA, Lee SM, et al. Dissociation of cerebral glucose metabolism and level of consciousness during the period of metabolic depression following human traumatic brain injury. *J Neurotrauma.* 2000; 17: 389–401.
13. Mehr SH, Gerdes SL. Medicolegal applications of PET scans. *NeuroRehabilitation.* 2001; 16(2): 87–92.
14. Rao N, Turski P, Polcyn E, Nickels RJ, Matthews CJ, Flynn MM. [18]F positron emission tomography in closed head injury. *Arch Phys Med Rehab.* 1984; 65: 780–785.
15. Dougall NJ, Bruggink S, Ebmeier KP. Systematic review of the diagnostic accuracy of 99mTc-HMPAO-SPECT in dementia. *Am J Geriatr Psychiatry.* 2004; 12(6): 554–570.
16. Castronovo FP, Jr. Technetium-99m: basic nuclear physics and chemical properties. *Am J Hosp Pharm.* 1975; 32(5): 480–488.
17. Appelbaum PS. Through a glass darkly: functional neuroimaging evidence enters the courtroom. *Psychiatric Services.* 2009; 60(1): 21–23.
18. Greely H, Illes J. Neuroscience-based lie detection: the urgent need for regulation. *Am J Law Med.* 2007; 33: 377–421.
19. Gurley JR, Marcus DK. The effects of neuroimaging and brain injury on insanity defenses. *Behav Sci Law.* 2008; 26: 85–97.

20. Fed. Rule Evid. 702 (2000).
21. *Daubert* v. *Merrell Dow Pharmaceuticals, Inc.*, 43 F.3d 1311 (9th Cir. 1995)
22. *Frye* v. *U.S.*, 293 F. 1013 (D.C. Cir.1923)
23. Brown E, Barglow P. Pseudocyesis. A paradigm for psychophysiological interactions. *Arch Gen Psychiatry.* 1971; 24: 221–229.
24. *California* v. *Miguel Carrizalez.* No. VCF 169926C Kelly-Frye hearing. Visalia, California. November 18–19, 2010. Reporter's transcript (1–267, at 261–262).
25. Weisberg DS, Keil FC, Goodstein J, Rawson E, Gray JR. The seductive allure of neuroscience explanations. *J Cog Neurosci.* 2008; 20(3): 470–477.
26. Brown T, Murphy E. Through a scanner darkly: functional neuroimaging as evidence of criminal defendant's past mental states. *Stanford Law Review.* 2010; 62: 1119–1208.
27. Schweitzer NS, Saks MJ, Murphy ER, Roskies AL, Sinnott-Armstrong W, Gaudet LM. Neuroimages as evidence in a *mens rea* defense: No impact. *Psychol Public Policy Law.* 2011; 17: 357–393.
28. *People* v. *Weinstein*, 591 N.Y.S.2d 715 (N.Y. Sup. 1992).
29. Rosen J. The brain on the stand. *New York Times.* March 11, 2007. Available online at http://www.nytimes.com/2007/03/11/magazine/11Neurolaw.t.html. Accessed March 31, 2014.
30. *Weinstein* v. *Dennison*, 801 N.Y.S.2d 244 (Sup. Ct. 2005).
31. Sneed C. Neuroimaging and the courts: standards and illustrative case index. *Emerging Issues in Neuroscience Conference for State and Federal Judges*: American Association for the Advancement of Science, the Federal Judicial Center, the National Center for State Courts, and the Dana Foundation; 2006.
32. Lasden M. Mr. Chiesa's brain—can hi-tech scans prove that criminal acts are the result of a damaged brain? *California Lawyer.* 2006; 26–30, 61–63.
33. MacLean A. Parole board denies Chiesa release plea. *The Union Demoncrat*, February 24, 2012. Available online at http://www.uniondemocrat.com/News/Local-News/Parole-board-denies-Chiesa-release-plea. Accessed March 31, 2014.
34. *Lockett* v. *Ohio*, 438 US 586 (1978).
35. *Tennard* v. *Dretke*, 542 U.S. 274 (2004).
36. *McKoy* v. *North Carolina*, 494 US 433 (1990).
37. *McCleskey* v. *Kemp*, 481 U.S. 279, 281 (1987).
38. *Strickland* v. *Washington*, 466 U.S. 668 (1984).
39. *Caro* v. *Calderon*, 165 F.3d 1223, 1228 (9th Cir.), cert. denied, 527 U.S. 1049, 119 S.Ct. 2414, 144 L.Ed.2d 811 (1999).
40. *Caro* v. *Woodford*, 280 F.3d 1247 (9th Cir.), cert. denied, 122 S. Ct. 2645 (2002).
41. *Smith* v. *Mullin*, 379 F.3d 919, Court of Appeals, 10th Circuit (2004).
42. *Hoskins* v. *State*, 702 So. 2d 202, 209 (Fla. 1997).
43. Fla. Stat. Ann. § 921.141 (1995).
44. *Hernandez* v. *Martel, Acting Warden, California State Prison at San Quentin*, 824 F.Supp.2d 1025 (2011).

CHAPTER 9

Chronic Traumatic Encephalopathy

MANISH A. FOZDAR AND HELEN M. FARRELL

Historically documented diseases sometimes have a resurgence. The increased incidence and prevalence of diseases such as tuberculosis and neurosyphilis in the Western Hemisphere after the HIV/AIDS epidemic are examples.[1] Harrison S. Martland, a pathologist from New Jersey, first described the syndrome of *dementia pugilistica* in boxers in his landmark 1928 *Journal of the American Medical Association* article.[2] He alluded to the considerable "head punishment" that boxers took and described various cognitive, neurologic, mood, and behavioral symptoms associated with this condition. Corsellis later identified the neuropathology of this syndrome in the brains of 15 deceased boxers, identifying several areas of brain damage.[3] He also described similar disease in other athletes with high risk of repetitive head injuries, such as jockeys and wrestlers. Critchley first used the term "chronic traumatic encephalopathy" (CTE) in his 1949 article.[4]

The high-profile suicides of several former National Football League (NFL) players and postmortem studies of their brains in recent years have drawn extraordinary attention to the topic of CTE.[5] These include former Chicago Bears safety Dave Duerson, who committed suicide by shooting himself in the chest so that his brain could be studied; it showed CTE.[6] This was followed by the suicide of Junior Seau, a 12-time Pro Bowler for the San Diego Chargers, who also shot himself. His brain has been studied at autopsy and shown to have CTE.[7,8] Resulting controversy has incorporated multiple areas of interest: medical, medicolegal, sociocultural, and sociopolitical. Lawsuits have been filed against the NFL, laws have been created at state and local levels, and fierce competition exists in medical academia to publish studies on the topic of CTE. This may affect how American football will be played several years down the road, especially considering the recent Centers for Disease Control and

Prevention (CDC) estimate of 1.6 to 3.8 million sports-related injuries occurring each year.[9]

SCOPE OF THE PROBLEM

Repetitive closed-head injuries, including concussion and subconcussion, have been described in multiple contact sports: football, boxing, wrestling, hockey, lacrosse, and soccer. In sports such as football, certain high-risk players sustain multiple (hundreds of) subconcussive hits per season.[10,11] Military veterans of modern warfare may be at high risk of developing CTE due to repeated exposure to blast-related concussions. The aforementioned high-profile suicides of several NFL players combined with the autopsy studies of their brains and careful neuropsychiatric and neurocognitive analysis of their lives prior to their death have thrust the subject of CTE to the forefront of the national psyche. Higher rates of neuropsychiatric and neurocognitive symptoms have been shown in retired contact-sport athletes compared to controls.[12-14] Multiple concussions are thought to be responsible for the development of CTE and hence the possibility of a dose-response relationship between the two.[13,14]

To understand the political, social, academic, and legal implications of the recent publicity on CTE, one needs to have a historical context. The NFL has received widespread criticism of its role in denying the problem of brain injury and its devastating effects on players. In a recent book, ESPN reporters thoroughly researched this issue.[15] The authors not only contend that NFL leadership willfully ignored the link between concussions sustained by the players and the subsequent development of multiple neurologic and neuropsychiatric symptoms, but also highlight the strong and often disrespectful differences of opinions among leading neuroscience researchers. Intense media publicity and lawsuits brought by former NFL players and their families have forced the league to alter its position—for example, by developing a protocol for players with concussion.[16]

The CDC's website documents extensively several policy and legislative changes that have taken place throughout the country at the local and state levels in an effort to increase awareness of and education about sports-related concussions.[17] Forty-three states and the District of Columbia have passed laws that govern return-to-play policies after an athlete has sustained a concussion.[17] The National Conference of State Legislatures has created online maps to track and update concussion-in-sports laws by state.[18]

CLINICAL PRESENTATION

Traumatic brain injury (TBI) is a very common problem that affects close to 1.7 million Americans each year and is a contributing factor in one third of injury-related deaths in the United States.[19] In addition to causing structural and behavioral problems, many TBI sufferers experience significant limitations in functions of daily living that lead to long-term disability.[20] Mild repetitive TBI can lead to the development of CTE, which is a progressive neurodegenerative condition associated with widespread deposition of tau protein in various parts of brain.[21] High-impact sports such as football, hockey, soccer, boxing, and wrestling are among the leading risk factors for CTE.[22]

Psychiatrists are frequently involved in cases of CTE due to the constellation of symptoms. Although there are no consensus-based clinical diagnostic criteria for CTE, the clinical syndrome of changes affects cognition, mood, personality, and movement. Omalu and colleagues[23] proposed common syndromal components of CTE based on their case series. Cognition is affected and manifests as problems with memory and executive functioning. Neuropsychological tests reliably show deficits in decision-making capacities, impulse control, problem solving, working memory, and mental flexibility.[12,24] Dementia occurs later in the disease.

Common mood problems include depression, apathy, libido changes, paranoia, aggression, hyperreligiosity, and suicidality. Personality and behavioral issues arise in the form of poor impulse control and behavioral disinhibition. Movement disorders include parkinsonism, gait disturbance, and other signs of motor neuron disease.[25]

Symptoms frequently begin with something as benign as a headache and progress to mild changes in concentration in the early stages. Following these early-stage warning signs are depression, aggression, explosive anger, and short-term memory loss. McKee and colleagues have proposed four stages of CTE based on neuropathologic criteria and clinical symptoms.[21] The symptoms, however, do not always progress in a predictable and sequential manner, which makes premortem detection challenging.[26]

Aggression can be externally or internally directed. External aggression often manifests with verbal outbursts and physical violence; internal aggression is self-directed and characteristic of suicide.[6,27,28] Behavioral dyscontrol has been defined as agitation, restlessness, impulsivity, disinhibition, irritability, lability, or explosive behavior.[24] CTE differs from acute concussion, postconcussive syndrome, or TBI in that the symptoms present years after the events occur; it is also pathologically distinctive.[26]

NEUROPATHOLOGY, NEUROANATOMY, AND NEUROCHEMISTRY OF CTE

The definitive diagnosis of CTE is made postmortem. A full autopsy must be performed with histochemical and immunohistochemical analyses of the brain to identify the presence of neurofibrillary tangles and neuritic threads. Structural, microscopic, and neurotransmitter dysfunction, however, can all contribute to the neuropathology of CTE.[28] There is often pronounced atrophy of the thalamus, hypothalamus, and mammillary bodies and pallor of the substantia nigra and locus coeruleus.[28] Microscopically, CTE is a neuropathologically distinct, slowly progressive tauopathy. There is prominent tau protein distributed in patches throughout the neocortex, distinguished from the diffuse amyloidosis following single-incident TBI. The advanced stages of CTE are accompanied by generalized atrophy of the brain with reduced brain weight, enlargement of the lateral and third ventricles, thinning of the corpus callosum, fenestrations in the cavum septum pellucidum, and scarring and neuronal loss of the cerebellar tonsils.[21] McKee and colleagues described the distinctive neuropathologic diagnostic criteria for CTE in a series of 85 cases of postmortem brain studies of former athletes, military veterans, and civilians with a history of repetitive mild TBI.[21]

The frontal lobes play a crucial role in executive cognitive processes and the regulation of emotion and behavior. The anterior frontal or prefrontal cortical areas subserving these functions are organized into five discrete but parallel and reciprocally interactive frontal-subcortical circuits: the premotor subcortical circuit, involved in the organization of voluntary motor function; the frontal eye field subcortical circuit, which facilitates voluntary eye movements; the anterior cingulate subcortical circuit, which subserves motivation and aspects of attention; the dorsolateral prefrontal cortex, which is responsible for executive functions; and the lateral orbitofrontal cortex, which modifies social intelligence.[29]

The dorsolateral prefrontal cortex is responsible for retrieving, categorizing, organizing, and sequencing information, problem solving, abstraction, judgment, and insight. These executive functions allow autonomous behavior and decrease behavioral dependency on environmental contingencies. The lateral orbitofrontal cortex appears to play a key role in suppressing aggression by supporting prosocial behavior, imbuing limbically driven appetites and emotions with social insight and judgment, and limiting contextually inappropriate, limbically driven behavioral responses.[30]

Suicidal ideation and attempts can occur with CTE. The risk for suicide, suicide attempts, and suicide ideation is increased in TBI survivors compared with the general population, even after adjustment for psychiatric comorbidities.[31] The National Institute of Mental Health Epidemiologic Catchment Area Program identified a higher frequency of suicide attempts in individuals with a history of TBI compared with those without (8.1 v. 1.9%).[32] Trauma-induced ventral frontal injury is associated with aggressive behavior, and since aggression may be either externally or internally directed, it is plausible that TBI survivors with injuries involving the lateral orbitofrontal cortex and its connections to other behaviorally salient neural networks may be at increased risk for suicidal behavior.[30]

Since aggression is a common sign of CTE, it is important to understand the neuroanatomy of aggression, especially in preparation for court testimony. The frontotemporal regions are particularly susceptible to the injurious effects of contact and inertial forces to which the brain is subjected during biomechanical trauma.[33,34] Shearing and straining forces damage white matter found in the brainstem, corpus callosum, and cerebral cortex.[35] Not only are brain structures affected by CTE, but major modulatory neurotransmitter systems (cholinergic, dopaminergic, noradrenergic, and serotonergic) projections are also affected.[36] These combinations of structural and neurochemical changes increase the likelihood of clinically significant early and late posttraumatic disturbances in cognition, emotion, and behavior.[30]

IN VIVO DIAGNOSIS OF CTE

At present there are no available in vivo biomarkers for the diagnosis of CTE. Definitive diagnosis is only through postmortem microscopic brain tissue examination. Although significant decreases in ApoE and Aβ concentrations in cerebrospinal fluid may correlate with the severity of the injury after TBI, there have been no similar studies in CTE. Advances in neuroimaging offer the promise of detecting subtle changes in axonal integrity in acute TBI and CTE. Standard T1- or T2-weighted structural magnetic resonance imaging (MRI) is helpful for quantitating pathology in acute TBI, but diffusion tensor MRI (DTI) is a more sensitive method to assess axonal integrity in vivo. In chronic moderate to severe TBI, abnormalities on DTI have been reported in the absence of observable lesions on standard structural MRI.[26] More severe white matter abnormalities on DTI have been associated with greater cognitive deficits by neuropsychological testing. Increases in whole-brain apparent diffusion coefficient and decreases in fractional anisotropy using DTI have been found in boxers compared to controls.

A recent study examined the presence of tau protein deposits in the brains of five living retired NFL athletes with histories of mood and cognitive problems.[37] This study utilized a tau tracer called 2-(1-{6-[(2-[F-18]fluoroethyl)(methyl)amino]-2-naphthyl}ethylidene)malononitrile (FDDNP) to detect tau deposits using positron emission tomography. Higher numbers of FDDNP signals were found in players compared with controls in the subcortical regions and amygdala. Binding values of FDDNP were higher in players with more concussions. The binding pattern was also consistent with the tau deposits pattern found in autopsy studies of CTE. The authors outlined the limitations of the study and suggested that this was a first step to guide future studies for in vivo detection of CTE neuropathology.

Researchers from Western Ontario University and Imperial College in London studied brain activity of 13 retired football players in comparison to 60 healthy subjects.[38] This was another in vivo study that used functional brain imaging technique. Subjects were asked to perform a standardized mental task (Stockings of Cambridge) while undergoing brain imaging. The brains of the former NFL players showed increased activity in the dorsolateral prefrontal cortex compared to control subjects. The researchers suggest that the NFL players' brains had to exert more effort to perform the same task and had to recruit "cognitive reserve" from other brain areas compared to normal subjects. Finally, the researchers suggest that the consistent changes observed in serially concussed brains of former NFL players may be an impending sign of more severe cognitive deficits that may emerge later in life.

CTE AND *DSM-5*

On May 18, 2013, the American Psychiatric Association published the 5th edition of the *Diagnostic and Statistical Manual of Mental Disorders*.[39] According to *DSM-5*, major clinical syndromal presentations of CTE could be diagnosed as shown in Table 9.1. Comorbid conditions may be present with

Clinical Presentation of CTE	*DSM-5* Diagnosis	ICD-9-CM Code (ICD-10-CM Code)*
Dementia and other cognitive disorders	*Major Neurocognitive Disorder Due to Traumatic Brain Injury*	
	(1) With Behavioral Disturbances	294.11 (F02.81)
	(2) Without Behavioral Disturbances	294.10 (F02.80)
	Minor Neurocognitive Disorder Due to Traumatic Brain Injury	331.83 (G31.84)
Personality change causing apathy, aggression, and disinhibition	*Personality Change Due to Another Medical Condition*	310.1 (F07.0)
Depression	*Depressive Disorder Due to Another Medical Condition*	293.83 (F06.31, F06.32, F06.34)
Legal involvement	*Problems Related to Crime or Interaction With the Legal System*	Various "v" codes V62.5, V62.89

Table 9.1. DIAGNOSES RELEVANT TO CTE

* ICD-10-CM codes effective October 1, 2014.

CTE and should be diagnosed as such (e.g., substance abuse, seizure disorder, and movement disorders [Parkinson disease, motor neuron disease]).

CTE, THE NFL, AND LAWSUITS

More than 3,000 retired NFL players or their relatives filed a class-action lawsuit against the NFL seeking compensation for having suffered from the effects of multiple concussions as a result of their participation in NFL games.[40] This lawsuit combined 80 separate tort claims filed against the NFL, and the master complaint, filed in federal court in Philadelphia, alleged that the NFL knowingly concealed information regarding the effects of repetitive concussions on players' brains and hence was negligent.[41] Korngold and colleagues discussed the substance of this master complaint and the resulting back-and-forth legal actions between the NFL and its insurers.[42] This lawsuit was tentatively settled on August 29, 2013, for $765 million, pending approval by the federal judge.[43] On January 14, 2014, U.S. District Court Judge Anita Brody denied the motion for preliminary approval and class certification without prejudice.[44] Her opinion expressed concerns about the fairness, reasonableness, and adequacy of the settlement and that the funds were insufficient to cover the future medical needs of the players.

Two other issues likely to play a role in future lawsuits against the NFL by players are worth mentioning. The Korngold group[42] argued that if courts rule in favor of the NFL by opining that its players are employees and hence covered under workers' compensation, then they would not be able to bring tort claims against the NFL, as employer negligence is not an element of such claims. Workers' compensation provides for medical coverage, a percentage of lost wages or salary, costs of rehabilitation and retraining, and payment for any permanent injury (usually based on an evaluation of limitation).[45] Disputes are resolved via a system of hearings and quasijudicial determinations by administrative law judges and appeal boards. Injured workers relinquish the right to sue for general damages (pain and suffering). This tradeoff is known as "the compensation bargain."

Another potential issue involves informed consent. Informed consent is an agreement to do something or to allow something to happen only after all the relevant and material facts and risks are known.[46] In contracts, an agreement may be reached only if there has been full disclosure by both parties of everything each party knows to be significant to the agreement. If NFL player contracts include full disclosure of the risks of repetitive brain injuries (concussions) and informed consent is obtained from the players at the time of signing the contract, then it may preclude future tort claims by players against the NFL.

In recent years, the NFL has taken steps to make the game safer by changing rules, having independent medical doctors examine players, and improving the testing and treatment of concussions.[47] It has donated millions of dollars toward research and education on brain injury. Whether the recent class-action settlement and positive changes implemented by NFL will reduce the threat of any major lawsuits in the future remains to be seen.

Within one week of the $765 million tentative settlement, four other former NFL players and their spouses filed a federal lawsuit in New Orleans against the NFL and its helmet maker, Riddell, Inc.[48] The plaintiffs alleged that they sustained one or more brain injuries and were suffering from headaches, dizziness, depression, memory loss, and confusion. As with earlier lawsuits, these plaintiffs also alleged that the NFL and its helmet maker failed to protect them from brain injuries. They demanded that the NFL and Riddell set up and fund medical monitoring and treatment programs for all former, current, and future NFL players. It will be quite some time before the outcome of this lawsuit is known. Expert testimony will be required on both sides to address the questions of causality and disability. Without neuropathology, however, the forensic examinations will have to be based on clinical profiles and syndromal presentations and on evolving brain-scanning technologies.

Ten former National Hockey League (NHL) players filed a class-action lawsuit against the league in November 2013.[49] The allegations and language of the complaint are similar to those of the NFL class-action lawsuit. The claim alleges that many NHL players suffer from the effects of repetitive concussions, leading to memory problems, depression, sleep problems, and other illnesses. It further alleges that the NHL knowingly concealed the severe risks of brain injury and encouraged the culture of violence.

CTE AND DISABILITY

The case of *Atkins v. Bert Bell/Pete Rozelle NFL Player Retirement Plan*[50] illustrates several issues that testifying medical experts may face in cases where CTE is alleged. The NFL Player Retirement Plan provides monthly Total & Permanent (T&P) disability benefits to eligible players. Players may be eligible for either of two types of T&P benefits: "Football Degenerative" or "Inactive." Disability arising out of NFL activities qualifies for "Football Degenerative" T&P benefits. Disability arising out of other causes qualifies for "Inactive" T&P benefits. "Football Degenerative" T&P benefits are significantly greater than "Inactive" T&P benefits. Each player's disability claim is initially reviewed by the Disability Initial Claims Committee. The Committee's decision can be appealed to the Retirement Board. The matter can be further referred to a Medical Advisory Physician to sort out medical issues, and the Retirement Board has the authority to refer disputed cases for final and binding arbitration. The claimants will want expert testimony to conclude that the injuries alleged had their genesis in playing football ("Football Degenerative"), whereas the defendants will rely on the ambiguity of the clinical syndromes and lack of neuropathologic "fingerprints" to suggest "Inactive" status.

Gene Atkins played professional football from 1987 to 1996. He was known as a hard-hitting and aggressive defensive back, sustaining a number of injuries in collisions with other players on the field. He filed a T&P disability application with the Plan administrators in December 2004, claiming that he suffered from chronic right shoulder pain and movement limitations, chronic neck pain with radiation to arms and hands, as well as depression and mood issues as a result of his chronic pain and functional limitations. He claimed that all his limitations resulted from playing football.

A neutral psychiatrist and a neutral orthopedist evaluated Atkins. The psychiatrist reported that he suffered from poor cognitive functioning but could not determine whether it resulted from playing football. The psychiatrist, however, found him totally disabled due to chronic pain, headaches, and neurologic defects. The orthopedist determined that Atkins did have neck and shoulder impairments as a result of playing football, but the impairments did not cause him to be totally disabled. The Disability Initial Claims Committee reviewed Atkins' application and specialist reports on June 7, 2005; his claim was denied.

A string of appeals and examinations by several medical providers followed over the next few years. Atkins was evaluated by another orthopedist, a neurologist, and then a neuropsychologist. The neurologist concluded that Atkins had a combination of impairments but his memory problems were not caused by playing football. The neuropsychologist concluded that Atkins had borderline intellectual functioning and was illiterate, neither of which was the result of playing football. He further opined that Atkins' main problems were psychiatric and due to his limited intelligence and resulting psychosocial disadvantages.

After reviewing all the above evidence, the Retirement Board granted Atkins Inactive T&P benefits for psychiatric impairments and decided that he did not qualify for Football Degenerative T&P benefits. This meant that he would receive substantially lower disability benefits. Atkins appealed to the Retirement Board to reclassify his benefits as Football Degenerative. Another neurologic examination was conducted by a different neurologist, who opined that he was suffering from multiple physical impairments due to his playing football but that he was not totally disabled. Accordingly, his request for reclassification was denied.

Following this denial, Atkins saw a neurosurgeon considered an authority on sports-related TBI and CTE. After examining Atkins the doctor opined that he suffered from severe postconcussive syndrome and probably early stages of CTE. He also opined that the claimant was totally disabled due to a "demented mental status." Atkins submitted this report to the Retirement Board and requested reconsideration and reclassification. The Disability Initial Claims Committee denied the request.

A few months later, Atkins received a favorable decision from the Social Security Administration and was awarded full Social Security Disability benefits dating to 1998. The Administrative Law Judge relied on the above-mentioned neurosurgeon's report along with another neurologist's report. After receiving the Social Security Administration's decision, Atkins reappealed to the Disability Initial Claims Committee. He was examined by yet another neutral neurologist, who opined that he suffered from cognitive deficits, chronic headaches, and depression and that only his headaches were due to playing football. He opined that cognitive deficits and depression were only partly the result of playing football.

Atkins filed a lawsuit against the Plan in federal district court. The suit was ultimately dismissed without prejudice. The Retirement Board referred the matter for final and binding arbitration. The arbitrator reviewed about 4,000 pages of records and opined that there was insufficient evidence to allow reclassification of Atkins' T&P benefits from Inactive to Football Degenerative. During the arbitration proceedings, the neurosurgeon/ CTE expert testified in his deposition that, based on his examination of Atkins, he had a high index of suspicion that Atkins suffered from CTE. He also stated that he could *not* say with scientific certainty that Atkins had CTE and that he could only know after examining his brain under the microscope.

Atkins appealed to the district court again, which granted summary judgment for the Plan, denying his request. He then appealed to U.S. Court of Appeals for the Fifth Circuit. This court affirmed the district court's granting of summary judgment in favor of the Plan.

CTE IN SOLDIERS AND VETERANS

TBI has been called "signature injury" of the Iraq and Afghanistan wars. One of the most common causes of TBI in this population is blast exposure from improvised explosive devices. Literature in this area is still emerging. One study looked at a brain autopsy on a 27-year-old Iraq war veteran who committed suicide by hanging.[51] The authors described findings consistent with CTE and similar to those found in football players. Goldstein and colleagues examined postmortem brains of four military veterans who were exposed to blast and/or concussive injuries. They also found evidence of CTE on neuropathologic examination.[52]

Many soldiers from these wars have returned home and are filing for disability and other veterans' benefits based on TBI claims. The U.S. Department of Veterans Affairs has expanded benefits for TBI and certain TBI-related conditions.[53] The Department of Veterans Affairs is overwhelmed with an increased caseload, and sociopolitical pressure has added urgency. Therefore, the Veterans Health Administration and Department of Defense are contracting with private providers to examine the veterans' disability claims. More and more civilian psychiatrists are likely to examine these claims.

POTENTIAL NEUROSCIENCE AND NEUROPSYCHIATRIC TESTIMONY IN CTE CASES

It is fair to say that neuroscience testimony is commonplace in courtrooms across the country. Between 2003 and 2013, the number of scientific publications in the "neurolaw" field has increased by more than 10 times.[54] Since 1993, all U.S. federal courts have applied Federal Rule of Evidence 702 (the *Daubert* standard) to determine the admissibility of scientific evidence.[55] Under Rule 702, the court, serving as gatekeeper, may rule on whether the proposed testimony has scientific support and literature, and whether its probative value outweighs the danger of prejudicing the jury (see Chapter 1). Many state courts continue to use the *Frye* standard, which requires that scientific testimony have general acceptance among its practitioners.[56]

Jones and colleagues provide useful and practical guidelines for neuroscientists who may testify as expert witnesses.[54] They assert that neuroscientists play a crucial role in helping judges and juries understand complex evidence and hence "separate wheat from chaff." Neuroscientists may also become secondary gatekeepers to help the court screen out dubious science. This determination is often made in a pretrial evidentiary hearing.

Due to the complex and evolving neuroscience involved in a potential legal case alleging CTE, we advise that testifying experts have comprehensive knowledge and experience. A psychiatrist asked to serve as an expert must first undertake an honest inventory of his or her skills: knowledge of brain injury, experience in evaluating and treating brain injury cases, familiarity with various neuroimaging techniques, thorough understanding of brain anatomy and brain–behavior relationships, neurocognitive assessment, and familiarity with recent scientific literature on CTE. A neuropsychiatrist/ behavioral neurologist is usually well equipped in these areas. Other areas of expertise likely to play a role, depending on the type of case, include neuroradiology, neuropathology, neuropsychology, neurology, and kinesiology. Table 9.2 highlights issues that a testifying neuropsychiatrist may plausibly encounter in a case of alleged CTE.

Table 9.2. TYPES OF CIVIL AND CRIMINAL LITIGATION INVOLVING CTE

Civil Cases	Criminal Cases
Neuropsychiatric symptoms: depression, behavioral/personality change, dementia	Behavioral dyscontrol due to CTE caused a person to commit the crime (diminished capacity defense)
Completed suicide	Cognitive changes due to CTE made the person unable to fully comprehend the financial transaction and hence not responsible for fraud.
Long-term disability	Cognitive deficits made the person incompetent to stand trial
Lost wages and loss of future earnings	Alleged CTE as a mitigating factor against severe punishment, including the death penalty
Testamentary capacity	Not guilty by reason of insanity (NGRI) defense
Wrongful death	

KEY POINTS FOR POTENTIAL EXPERT WITNESSES

Evaluating neuropsychiatrists should keep in mind the following clinical considerations while serving as an expert in CTE cases:[42]

1. CTE cannot be confirmed as a diagnosis until a microscopic examination of the brain is performed. The closest to in vivo diagnostic certainty is "probable CTE," similar to an Alzheimer disease diagnosis.
2. Causal relationships of repetitive concussions and mild TBI with subsequent behavioral symptoms may not be clear, due to a delay in the onset of neurologic signs and symptoms after initial traumas.
3. No clear dose–response relationship (number of concussions and subsequent severity of symptoms) has been established in football. The witness should be up to date regarding research in this area.
4. A comprehensive neuropsychiatric evaluation must be undertaken, including detailed medical, psychiatric, substance abuse, developmental, family, and psychosocial histories. In living ex-players, no evaluation is complete without a thorough physical examination, especially a neurologic one.
5. The examiner must be familiar with the diagnostic tests necessary to support the diagnosis. Examples include relevant neuroimaging modalities, neuropsychological tests, and blood tests (including genetic tests when relevant).
6. The examiner must be familiar with common syndromal presentations of CTE.
7. Extra caution should be exercised on the part of the examiner to remain objective in light of the high publicity in many of these cases. To that

end, potential confounding factors should be investigated thoroughly, including substance abuse, availability of a psychosocial support system, developmental history, prior criminal record, and other medical conditions.

8. The examining forensic psychiatrist should consider working in concert with other experts, such as a neuropathologist, neuroradiologist, and neuropsychologist.

APPLICATIONS

A psychiatrist may be asked either by plaintiff's or defendant's counsel to evaluate a claimant who is applying for disability benefits on the basis of CTE. As we saw in the case of Atkins, such a claim can be vigorously contested. Psychiatric testimony may also be required in a wrongful-death lawsuit where the estate of a suicide victim alleges a causal link between CTE and suicide. The establishment of a diagnosis is aided by a neuropathology report, although the basis for the association between CTE and suicide is not fully described.

In disability cases, the first order of business for the evaluating psychiatrist should be to establish a detailed concussion history by examining the claimant, interviewing collateral informants, and reviewing available documents such as NFL game records, military records, and medical records. Considering that in vivo diagnostic tools for CTE are still in the very early stages of development, the onus is on the evaluating psychiatrist to gather enough information that can support or refute the *probable* diagnosis of CTE. Then there is a question of how to apportion *causality*. That is, in the case of most contact sports, the players' careers began in childhood, not upon joining a professional league. As we saw in Chapter 4, early insults to the brain may lead to sustained changes that become apparent only in adulthood. Accordingly, expert witnesses are cautioned not to disregard the effects of repeated TBI throughout the life course of an athlete. This complication is usually less troublesome in the case of soldiers with blast-injury claims, as the exposure is time-limited and better documented.

The Atkins case echoes the fierce disagreements that exist in academia over CTE as a diagnostic entity and its causal link to any neurocognitive and neurobehavioral disorders. Therefore, it is safe to assume that, based on the same information, there may be two or more differing opinions from different experts. Because the subject matter is complex and unfamiliar to jurors, the court will need to decide (e.g., at a *Daubert* hearing) who can testify and what can be said.

Experts must also be able to offer and discuss differential diagnostic considerations. For example, in a case of a wrongful-death claim involving suicide, multiple risk factors may be present in the history of the deceased: previous history of substance abuse, family history of depression and suicide, and personal history of impulsivity that may predate the documented history of concussions. If the examining psychiatrist concludes that CTE was a significant contributing factor to the depression and suicide of the claimant, the report should reflect the basis for the opinion and whether other risk factors or explanations were considered. While the pathophysiology of suicide is not within the purview of this discussion, it is important to remember that suicide is a complex behavior shaped by the convergence of multiple factors, including developmental, psychosocial, biologic, and genetic ones. No single factor can be asserted as a sole causal link to such a complex behavior. CTE can be a substantial contributing factor in suicidal behavior via neurobiologic changes, depression, and psychosocial factors. Therefore, a plaintiff's expert may be able to opine that CTE was *a* proximate cause of suicide or CTE was *more than likely a significant contributing factor* leading to suicidal behavior. This is assuming the proposed testimony has survived any evidentiary challenges. The defense expert may correctly counter that the causal link between CTE and suicide is *terra incognita* and that testimony on the subject amounts only to speculation.

Evaluation of a claimant who is applying for disability on the basis of alleged CTE diagnosis should also follow the above general guidelines. The expert's report should include an analysis of premorbid and current clinical data. A conclusion that a purported syndromal presentation of depression, behavioral changes, and cognitive impairment represents CTE should be weighed against clinical evidence of preexisting as well as coexisting confounding factors. Taking our cues again from the Atkins case, experts should never glibly attribute a syndrome to a specific neuropsychiatric disorder. All conclusions must be stated within reasonable medical certainty and supportable through available data and, where applicable, published research.

Assessment of any neurocognitive impairment in someone with possible CTE must start with systematic collection of developmental data, school records, any possible psychological/neuropsychological evaluations done in school or college, collateral information from relatives and other associates, detailed medical and psychiatric histories, substance abuse history, and a thorough history of concussions when available. Comprehensive neuropsychological testing must include effort and validity testing as well as personality tests. Written reports should describe the findings of neuropsychological testing in the full context of other available data.

Any type of neuroimaging evidence introduced by the expert must meet the evidentiary standards and, in *Daubert* jurisdictions particularly, its probative value should outweigh any potential biases it may introduce in the courtroom. Baugh and colleagues[26] discuss possible uses of various structural and functional neuroimaging techniques in CTE. If functional neuroimaging such as a positron emission tomogram scan is ordered as part of the evaluation process, any reported abnormality must be interpreted with caution and may not be indicative of brain trauma.[57] More important, scientific evidence is too weak to link any positron emission tomogram scan abnormality to abnormal behavior.[57]

Criminal defendants may assert an insanity or a diminished capacity defense on the basis of neurobehavioral and neurocognitive impairments allegedly due to CTE. Due to relaxed evidentiary standards in the penalty phase of the trial compared to the guilt/innocence phase, a CTE-related defense is more likely to be successful in mitigation (penalty phase) versus exculpation (guilt phase).

CONCLUSIONS

While CTE is not a recently discovered clinical diagnostic entity, it is fair to say that never before has it received so much attention so quickly. Various factors converged at the right time within the past few years to draw extraordinary attention to this topic: the willingness of deceased NFL players' families to donate brains for postmortem study, the availability of advanced medical techniques to study those brains, the application of knowledge gained in other areas of neuroscience to the subject of CTE, the class-action lawsuit filed by former NFL players, and intense media coverage of the topic.

Postmortem brain studies of deceased NFL players have consistently demonstrated unique neuropathologic findings that define CTE. While a definitive diagnosis of CTE remains a postmortem diagnosis, research is well under way to study CTE in vivo. This research heavily relies on various neuroimaging protocols. As it becomes more refined, more reliable and consistent criteria may emerge that may establish the diagnosis of CTE in vivo. In view of this reality, testifying experts should follow the guidelines mentioned above while evaluating a case of potential CTE and offering testimony.

REFERENCES

1. Sharma SK, Mohan A. Tuberculosis: from an incurable scourge to a curable disease—journey over a millennium. *Indian J Med Res.* 2013; 137(3): 455–493.
2. Martland HS. Punch drunk. *JAMA.* 1928; 91: 1103–1107.
3. Corsellis JA, Bruton CJ, Freeman-Browne D. The aftermath of boxing. *Psychol Med.* 1973; 3: 270–303.
4. Critchley M. Punch-drunk syndromes: the chronic traumatic encephalopathy of boxers. In Verbiest H, ed. *Hommage á Clovis Vincent.* Paris: Maloine; 1949.

5. Cantu RC. Chronic traumatic encephalopathy in the National Football League. *Neurosurgery*. 2007; 61(2): 223–225. doi: 10.1227/01.NEU.0000255514.73967.90

6. Schwarz A. Duerson's brain trauma diagnosed. *New York Times*, May 2, 2011. Available online at http://www.nytimes.com/2011/05/03/sports/football/03duerson.html. Accessed October 5, 2013.

7. ESPN.com News Services. Junior Seau's death ruled a suicide. May 2, 2012. Available online at http://espn.go.com/nfl/story/_/id/7888037/san-diego-county-medical-examiner-office-rules-junior-seau-death-suicide. Accessed October 5, 2013.

8. ESPN.com news services. Junior Seau family: brain study OK. May 4, 2012. Available online at http://espn.go.com/nfl/story/_/id/7889467/junior-seau-family-allow-concussion-study-brain. Accessed October 5, 2013.

9. Centers for Disease Control and Prevention. National Center for Injury Prevention and Control. Nonfatal traumatic brain injuries from sports and recreation activities—United States, 2001–2005. *MMWR Weekly*. 2007; 56(29): 733–737.

10. Beckwith JG, Chu JJ, Greenwald RM. Validation of a noninvasive system for measuring head acceleration for use during boxing competition. *J Appl Biomech*. 2007; 23: 238–244.

11. Greenwald RM, Gwin JT, Chu JJ, Crisco JJ. Head impact severity measures for evaluating mild traumatic brain injury risk exposure. *Neurosurgery*. 2008; 62: 789–798.

12. Wall SE, Williams WH, Cartwright-Hatton S, et al. Neuropsychological dysfunction following repeat concussions in jockeys. *J Neurol Neurosurg Psychiatry*. 2006; 77: 518–520.

13. Guskiewicz KM, Marshall SW, Bailes JE. Association between recurrent concussion and late-life cognitive impairment in retired professional football players. *Neurosurgery*. 2005; 57: 719–726.

14. Guskiewicz KM, Marshall SW, Bailes JE, et al. Recurrent concussion and risk of depression in retired professional football players. *Med Sci Sports Exerc*. 2007; 39: 903–909.

15. Fainaru-Wada M, Fainaru S. *League of Denial: The NFL, Concussions and the Battle for Truth*. New York: Crown Archetype; 2013.

16. NFL's 2013 protocol for players with concussion. October 1, 2013. Available online at http://www.nflevolution.com/article/nfl%27s-2013-protocol-for-players-with-concussions?ref=0ap2000000253716. Accessed October 2, 2013.

17. Injury Prevention & Control: Traumatic Brain Injury. Available online at http://www.cdc.gov/concussion/policies.html Last reviewed March 14, 2013. Last updated September 26, 2013. Accessed October 5, 2013.

18. Map of Concussion in Sports Legislation. National Conference of State Legislatures. Available online at http://www.ncsl.org/issues-research/health/traumatic-brain-injury-legislation.aspx. Updated July 2013, Accessed October 5, 2013.

19. Centers for Disease Control and Prevention. How many people have TBI? Available online at http://www.cdc.gov/TraumaticBrainInjury/statistics.html Last reviewed March 18, 2013. Last updated March 27, 2013. Accessed October 5, 2013.

20. Selassie AW, Zaloshnja E, Langlois JA, Miller T, Jones P, Steiner C. Incidence of long-term disability following traumatic brain injury hospitalization, United States, 2003. *J Head Trauma Rehabil*. 2008; 23: 123–131.

21. McKee AC, Stein TD, Nowinski CJ, et al. The spectrum of disease in chronic traumatic encephalopathy. *Brain.* 2013; 136; 43–64. doi:10.1093/brain/aws307

22. Gavett BE, Stern RA, McKee AC. Chronic traumatic encephalopathy: a potential late effect of sport-related concussive and subconcussive head trauma. *Clin Sports Med.* 2011; 30(1): 179–188.

23. Omalu BI, Hamilton RL, Kamboh MI, DeKosky ST, Bailes J. Chronic traumatic encephalopathy (CTE) in a National Football League player: case report and emerging medicolegal practice questions. *J Foren Nurs.* 2010; 6: 40–46. doi: 10.1111/j.1939-3938.2009.01064.x

24. Collins MW, Grindel SH, Lovell MR, et al. Relationship between concussion and neuropsychological performance in college football players. *JAMA.* 1999; 282: 964–970.

25. Gavett BE, Cantu RC, Shenton, et al. Clinical appraisal of chronic traumatic encephalopathy: current perspectives and future directions. *Curr Op Neurol.* 2011; 24: 525–531.

26. Baugh CM, Stamm JM, Riley DO, et al. Chronic traumatic encephalopathy: neurodegeneration following repetitive concussive and subconcussive brain trauma. *Brain Imaging Behav.* 2012; 6(2): 244–254. doi: 10.1007/s11682-012-9164-5.

27. Omalu BI, Bailes J, Hammers JL, Fitzsimmons RP. Chronic traumatic encephalopathy, suicides and parasuicides in professional American athletes: the role of the forensic pathologist. *Am J Foren Med Pathol.* 2010; 31(2): 130–132.

28. McKee AC, Cantu RC, Nowinski CJ. Chronic traumatic encephalopathy in athletes: progressive tauopathy after repetitive head injury. *J Neuropathol Exp Neurol.* 2009; 68(7): 709–735.

29. Wortzel H, Arcinegas D. A forensic neuropsychiatric approach to traumatic brain injury, aggression, and suicide. *J Am Acad Psychiatry Law.* 2013; 41: 274–286.

30. Mega MS, Cummings JL. Frontal-subcortical circuits and neuropsychiatric disorders. *J Neuropsychiatry Clin Neurosci.* 1994; 6: 358–370.

31. Simpson G, Tate R. Suicidality in people surviving a traumatic brain injury: prevalence, risk factors and implications for clinical management. *Brain Inj.* 2007; 21: 1335–1351.

32. Oquendo MA, Friedman JH, Grunebaum MF, Burke A, Silver JM, Mann JJ. Suicidal behavior and mild traumatic brain injury in major depression. *J Nerv Ment Dis.* 2004; 192: 430–434.

33. Bigler ED. Anterior and middle cranial fossa in traumatic brain injury: relevant neuroanatomy and neuropathology in the study of neuropsychological outcome. *Neuropsychology.* 2007; 21: 515–531.

34. Povlishock JT, Katz DI. Update of neuropathology and neurological recovery after traumatic brain injury. *J Head Trauma Rehabil.* 2005; 20: 76–94.

35. Meythaler JM, Peduzzi JD, Eleftheriou E, Novack TA. Current concepts: diffuse axonal injury-associated traumatic brain injury. *Arch Phys Med Rehabil.* 2001; 82: 1461–1471.

36. Arcinegas DB, Silver JM. Pharmacotherapy of post-traumatic cognitive impairments. *Behav Neurol.* 2006; 17: 25–42.

37. Small GW, Kepe V, Siddarth P, et al. PET scanning of brain tau in retired National Football League players: preliminary findings. *Am J Geriatr Psychiatry.* 2013; 21(2): 138–144.

38. Healy M. NFL players' brains at work show early signs of concussions' toll. *Los Angeles Times*, October 17, 2013. Available online at http://www.latimes.com/science/sciencenow/la-sci-nfl-brains-concussions-toll-20131016,0,7137694.story. Accessed October 18, 2013.

39. *Diagnostic and Statistical Manual of Mental Disorders*, 5th ed. Washington, DC: American Psychiatric Association; 2013.

40. Tierney M. Football player who killed himself had brain disease. *New York Times*, July 26, 2012. Available online at http://www.nytimes.com/2012/07/27/sports/football/ray-easterling-autopsy-found-signs-of-brain-disease-cte.html. Accessed October 9, 2013.

41. *Gerald Allen, Joseph Kowalewski, David Little, Shawn Wooden*, and Ron Fellows, *Original Class Action* v. *National Football League and NFL Properties*. No. 2:12-cv-03224-AB (E.D. Pa. 2012).

42. Korngold C, Farrell H, Fozdar M. The National Football League and chronic traumatic encephalopathy: legal implications. *J Am Acad Psychiatry Law*. 2013; 41: 430–436. Excerpt reprinted with permission from the American Academy of Psychiatry and the Law.

43. Boren C. NFL, ex-players reach settlement over concussion lawsuits. *The Washington Post* online, August 29, 2013. Available online at http://www.washingtonpost.com/blogs/early-lead/wp/2013/08/29/nfl-former-players-to-settle-concussion-lawsuits-judge-says/. Accessed October 9, 2013.

44. *In re: National Football League Players' Concussion Injury Litigation*. MDL No. 2323, 12-md-2323, Document 5657, P.1–12.

45. Ciccone JR, Jones JCW. Personal injury litigation and forensic psychiatric assessment. In Simon RI, Gold LH, eds. *The American Psychiatric Publishing Textbook of Forensic Psychiatry*, 2nd ed. Washington, DC: American Psychiatric Publishing, Inc., 2010: 260–301.

46. Knoll JL. Ethics in forensic psychiatry. In Simon RI, Gold LH, eds. *The American Psychiatric Publishing Textbook of Forensic Psychiatry*, 2nd ed. Washington, DC: American Psychiatric Publishing, Inc., 2010: 111–149.

47. Waldron T. What does the NFL's concussion settlement mean for the future of football? *Think Progress*, August 29, 2013. Available online at http://think-progress.org/sports/2013/08/29/2552921/nfls-concussion-settlement-mean-future-football/. Accessed October 11, 2013.

48. Associated Press. Four ex-NFL players file new concussion law suit against league. September 3, 2013. Available online at http://www.nfl.com/news/story/0ap1000000237961/article/four-exnfl-players-file-new-concussion-lawsuit-against-league. Accessed October 11, 2013.

49. Ex-Leafs Gary Leeman, Rick Vaive among 10 NHLers launching concussion lawsuit. Thestar.com, November 25, 2013. Available online at http://www.thestar.com/sports/hockey/2013/11/25/exleafs_gary_leeman_rick_vaive_among_10_nhlers_launching_concussion_lawsuit.html. Accessed January 25, 2014.

50. *Atkins* v. *Bert Bell/Pete Rozelle NFL Player Retirement Plan*, 694 F. 3d 557—U.S. Court of Appeals, 5th Circuit, 2012.

51. Omalu B, Hammers JL, Bailes J, et al. Chronic traumatic encephalopathy in an Iraqi war veteran with posttraumatic stress disorder who committed suicide. *Neurosurg Focus*. 2011; 31(5): E3.

52. Goldstein LE, Fisher AM, Tagge CA, et al. Chronic traumatic encephalopathy in blast-exposed military veterans and a blast neurotrauma mouse model. *Sci Transl Med.* 2012; 4, 134ra60. doi: 10.1126/scitranslmed.3003716.
53. VA to expand benefits for traumatic brain injury. December 16, 2013. Available online at Ihttp://www.va.gov/opa/pressrel/pressrelease.cfm?id=2506. Accessed on January 28, 2014.
54. Jones OD, Wagner AD, Faigman DL, Raichle ME. Neuroscientists in court. *Nature Reviews: Neuroscience.* 2013; 14: 730–736. doi:10.1038/nrn3585.
55. Rule 702 of Federal Rules of Evidence. December 1, 2010. Available online at http://www.uscourts.gov/uscourts/rulesandpolicies/rules/2010%20rules/evidence.pdf. Accessed October 14, 2013.
56. *Frye* v. *U.S.*, 293 F1013 (D. C. Cir. 1923).
57. Moriarty JC, Langleben DD, Provenzale JM. Brain trauma, PET scans and forensic complexity. *Behav Sci Law.* 2013. doi: 10.1002/bsl.

CHAPTER 10

Designer Drugs and Criminal Responsibility

SAMSON GURMU AND KENNETH J. WEISS*

Drug- and alcohol-related behaviors are among the most frequent encountered by mental health practitioners in clinical practice and forensic settings. Voluntary substance use, however, is rarely the basis of a defense to criminal charges and may in fact work against a defendant. The situation could be altered when novel (legal) substances are used or when a drug causes unintended or unexpected behavioral toxicity. In this chapter, we will explore the interaction of novel compounds and behavioral toxicity in the context of potential claims of diminished responsibility.

TRENDS IN SUBSTANCE USE

Psychiatric and physical sequelae of substance use constitute a major threat to public health. This is especially true when highly potent receptor-active drugs are released into the population, often starting as unregulated substances. Accordingly, several large-scale efforts quantify substance use patterns on a periodic basis. In the United States, 3 surveys are published annually: the National Survey on Drug Use and Health (NSDUH), a national-level community survey; Monitoring the Future (MTF), conducted on American adolescents and young adults; and the Drug Abuse Warning Network (DAWN), consisting of information on drug-related emergency department visits across the United States and drug-related deaths reported by medical examiners and

---

* Portions of this chapter were previously published as: Weiss KJ. 'Wet' and wild: PCP and criminal responsibility. *J Psychiatry Law.* 2004; 32: 361–384. Used with permission from Federal Legal Publications, Inc., Somers, NY.

coroners.[1-3] Most national and regional epidemiologic data regarding drug use in the United States come from these surveys. However, there is a dearth of information from these large surveys regarding new and emerging drugs.

According to the NSDUH, an estimated 22.5 million Americans over age 12 were current illicit drug users in 2011, representing 8.7% of the U.S. population in this age range.[1] There are no data, however, on new and emerging drugs of abuse. The first national survey to include synthetic cannabinoids (SCs) was the MTF survey of 2011, which found that 11.4% of high school seniors had used them, making synthetic cannabinoids the most widely used class of illicit drugs after marijuana itself.[3] SCs also appeared for the first time in the DAWN report in 2010, with 11,406 emergency room visits attributed to SCs.[2] By 2011, the number had reached 28,531 visits, a 150% increase.[2] On the other hand, the only reported data on synthetic cathinones ("bath salts") came from the 2012 MTF survey, which reported a 1.2% use prevalence among high school seniors.[3] Despite the absence of systematic data on bath salts use, some useful information can be gleaned from poison control centers data. In 2010 and 2011 respectively, there were 304 and 6,136 calls reported.[4] Data from the Drug Enforcement Administration (DEA) also indicate that bath salts have been encountered in every state and the District of Columbia.[5]

DESIGNER DRUGS

A designer drug, according to the Designer Drug Enforcement Act of 1986, is "a substance other than a controlled substance that has a chemical structure substantially similar to that of a controlled substance in schedule I or II or that was specifically designed to produce an effect substantially similar to that of a controlled substance in schedule I or II." Apparent in this definition is the lack of any physiologic specificity to the term "designer drug." Designer drugs include what are variously referred to as "new psychoactive substances," "legal highs," "herbal highs," "research chemicals," "laboratory agents," and "bath salts." Analogs of natural and synthetic opioid compounds, analogs of amphetamine and cathinone products, and SCs and phencyclidine (PCP) analogs are among the best-studied designer drugs manufactured by clandestine chemists. In this chapter we will restrict the discussion to forensic aspects of SCs and synthetic cathinone compounds.

DESIGNER DRUGS IN THE NEWS

The sensational story of "the Causeway face attacker" in Miami, who on May 26, 2012, assaulted and bit most of the face off his victim, catapulted bath salts into national attention.[6] While the attacker's toxicology was eventually declared negative for both synthetic cathinones and cannabinoids, the story highlighted the difficulty of capturing a single compound when the number of synthetic designer substances may be in the hundreds.[7]

The past few years have seen many accounts by law enforcement, emergency medical services, and poison control call centers of bizarre, erratic, and sometimes violent behavior following the use of designer drugs.[8] In March 2011, a Pennsylvania man with no serious drug history entered a monastery in Scranton and stabbed a priest. Before and during his trial, no clear motive for the act was disclosed. Then it was revealed that the young man was quite intoxicated at the time of arrest after a several-day binge on bath salts purchased from a local store.[9]

One winter night in 2010, a 21-year-old Louisiana man, high on the "Cloud 9" bath salts he had snorted, cut his throat in front of his father and his sister.[10] Having missed major vessels, he survived, only to kill himself with a .22-caliber youth rifle a few hours later.[10] The autopsy revealed the synthetic cathinone methylenedioxypyrovalerone (MDPV).[11] MDPV has also been implicated at autopsy in a case of murder-suicide from Washington state, where an Army medic shot his wife and himself in front of the police trooper who stopped him for speeding.[12]

Perhaps the most publicized case of an adverse reaction associated with use of SCs is that of a 19-year-old male from Illinois who, after having smoked the "herbal incense" iAroma, began experiencing severe panic attacks and started driving in an erratic manner at a high speed before fatally crashing into a home.[13] His toxicology revealed the presence of the SC JWH-210.[13]

REGULATORY RESPONSES

Serious efforts at regulating designer drugs date to the 1980s, when attempts to synthesize analogs of meperidine, then a tightly regulated opioid, resulted in toxic byproducts that caused irreversible symptoms of advanced parkinsonism.[14] These attempts to synthesize analogs reflected a desire by manufacturers and consumers to bypass the Controlled Substances Act of 1970 (CSA). The CSA individually lists dangerous drugs whereby possession, sale, and use were prohibited. In response, Congress enacted the Controlled Substance Analogue Enforcement Act of 1986 (Federal Analog Act).[15] As the name suggests, the law was meant to control "substantially similar" analogs of controlled substances that produce a similar effect, yet distinct enough to be designated as different chemical compounds.[15] However, the Federal Analog Act does not apply if the substance is "not intended for human consumption."[16] This loophole has been exploited by manufacturers, who prominently display the disclaimer on their packaging. Not surprisingly, both

CSA and the Federal Analog Act have failed to contain the rapid spread of SCs, synthetic bath salts, and other designer drugs.[14]

The traditional approach (CSA) of individually listing drugs one by one through legislation is far too bureaucratic and slow to catch up with the appearance of new drugs. The ability of the DEA to use emergency powers to temporarily schedule new substances to the list itself has been criticized as a slow and lengthy process.[14] The Federal Analog Act, on the other hand, has been challenged as being too vague and overly broad; specifically, attempts have been made to challenge the "substantially similar" and "intent" requirements.[17] Manufacturers have also exploited the intent requirement by selling "research chemicals," "incense," or "bath salts" that are labeled "not for human consumption." In 2011, the DEA temporarily scheduled 5 SCs and 3 synthetic cathinones using its emergency powers.[18] In light of the number and variety of these chemicals, this approach was easily circumvented by the manufacturers of the synthetic drugs.[19]

At the state level, efforts to control synthetic drugs were under way before the federal government instituted the emergency ban. State legislatures, like the federal government, use a combination of individual listings of drugs and analog acts. Some states, however, omit either the "substantial similarity" requirement found in federal law or the "intent" requirement to close loopholes used by distributors of designer drugs. Because states have fewer procedural requirements, individual listings of drugs have been more efficient than at the federal level.

The Synthetic Drug Abuse Prevention Act of 2012 (SDAPA), in addition to combining aspects of individual drug listings and analog (class) language, has attempted to predict analogs of a controlled substance (even those not yet distributed). It does so by using generic descriptions of important functional molecular components that could be modified to synthesize new variants. The DEA under the SDAPA also has expanded temporary scheduling powers to make enforcement more efficient.

"SPICE" AND OTHER SCS

SCs are potent cannabinoid-receptor agonists manufactured in clandestine labs that are packaged and sold as herbal products (e.g., incense) under a variety of brand names such as "Spice," "K2," "Black Mamba," "Yucatan Fire," and "Moon Rocks."[20,21] Spice products are typically advertised as medicinal herbs, but their psychoactive properties derive not from the "herbal" portion but from the synthetic chemicals sprayed onto dried plant material.[22] SCs were initially produced in research laboratories at pharmaceutical companies and academic centers. One such lab, headed by Professor John W. Huffman at Clemson University, after whom the JWH series of cannabinoids is named, has produced hundreds of SCs.[23]

Clinical Effects of SCs

The physiologic effects of SCs stem from their action at the cannabinoid-1 receptor (CB-1) in a fashion similar to the Δ^9-tetrahydrocannabinol (THC) found in marijuana.[21,24] Unlike natural marijuana, which contains several other psychoactive compounds that modulate the effect of THC, SCs tend to be chemically purer, with fewer constituents.[25] The net clinical and physiologic effects of cannabis correlate better with the ratio of its constituent components, specifically the ratio of THC to cannabidiol (CBD).[26,27] SCs, lacking CBD, which has antagonistic effects at the CB-1 receptor, represent an unmodulated stimulation of the CB-1 receptor. In addition they typically are much more potent than THC at the receptor level.[21] For example, JWH-018, one of the more widely used SCs, has a CB-1 affinity 5-fold that of THC.[28] An expert witness will want to be familiar with this disparity when explaining drug effects that are different from what is typical. Considering that there are several hundred SCs available and a large variety of products on the market with variable and inconsistent cannabinoid composition and potency, it may be difficult for the user to control or predict adverse consequences. Thus, from an expert witness' point of view, there is a question of whether the ultimate effects on the individual were *voluntary* or *involuntary*.

The most common acute adverse clinical effects are summarized in Table 10.1. Long-term effects of SC use have not been systematically studied.[28]

SYNTHETIC CATHINONES OR "BATH SALTS"

The term "bath salts" refers to several synthetic chemicals derived from cathinone.[29] In the United Kingdom and continental Europe, the terms "plant food" or "plant feeders" are also used to describe synthetic cathinones.[29] Cathinone is a natural alkaloid found in khat (*Catha edulis*), a shrub whose leaves are chewed or dried and consumed as tea for their stimulant properties in eastern Africa and the Arabian peninsula.[30] On the street, synthetic cathinones are sold under different brand names such as Bliss, Blizzard, Blue Silk, Cloud Nine, Drone, Ivory Snow, Ivory Wave, Ivory Coast, Pure Ivory, Purple Wave, Vanilla Sky, and White Rush.[29,31] While many cathinone analogs and derivatives have been used, the main ingredients appear to be mephedrone, methylone, or MDPV.[31] In Europe, where bath salts appeared earlier than in America, regulators have noted more than 30 synthetic cathinones as potential drugs of abuse.[29] Structural-functional analyses of cathinone and its derivatives reveal similarity not only with amphetamines but also with lysergic acid diethylamide (LSD).[30] As with SCs, the regulation of a cathinone compound is usually followed by the appearance of new derivatives on the market as "legal" alternatives for consumers.[32]

Table 10.1. SYNTHETIC CANNABINOIDS: ADVERSE CLINICAL EFFECTS

Central Nervous System	Psychosis
	Seizures
	Anxiety
	Agitation
	Irritability
	Memory changes
	Sedation
	Confusion
Cardiovascular	Tachycardia
	Arrhythmias
	Cardiotoxicity and chest pain
Gastrointestinal	Nausea and vomiting
Other	Appetite changes
	Tolerance, withdrawal and dependence (inner unrest, craving, nocturnal nightmares, sweating, headache and tremor)

Adapted from Seely KA, Lapoint J, Moran JH, Fattore L. Spice drugs are more than harmless herbal blends: a review of the pharmacology and toxicology of synthetic cannabinoids. *Progr Neuropsychopharmacol Biol Psychiatry.* 2012; 39(2): 234–243.[28]

Unlike SCs, which are almost always smoked, bath salts can be taken intranasally, swallowed, or injected. There have also been reports of bath salts being applied to the gums or inserted into the vagina or rectum.[31] Bath salts are noted for their stimulant effects (Table 10.2). Their clinical effects have been compared to other stimulants, such as methamphetamine.[33] However, it appears that the incidence of adverse neuropsychiatric effects is also quite high.[29,31,34] This could be due to structural attributes of synthetic cathinones that are shared with known hallucinogens such as LSD.[30] A recent study looking at bath-salt–related clinical information in the National Poison Control Center's data system for 9 states found that the most common clinical findings were agitation in about two thirds of cases and hallucinations in about one third.[34] The same study noted that benzodiazepines and antipsychotics were the most commonly used medications in bath-salts–related emergency department visits. To date there have not been any studies aimed at determining the long-term consequences of the use of bath salts.[31]

DESIGNER DRUGS AND VIOLENT CRIME

Use of substances with psychoactive properties has been associated with a variety of offenses, many violent. According to Department of Justice data, half of all adult probationers, one third of all state prisoners, and one quarter

Table 10.2. PHYSICAL AND NEUROPSYCHIATRIC EFFECTS OF BATH SALTS

	Desirable Effects	Adverse Effects
Physical	Alertness	Cerebral edema
	Analgesia	Diaphoresis
	Increased energy	Hyperreflexia
	Stimulation	Hypertension
		Hyperthermia
		Jaw tension
		Muscle spasm
		Mydriasis
		Myocardial infarction
		Respiratory distress
		Seizure
		Tachycardia
Neuropsychiatric	Creativity	Aggression
	Empathy	Violent behavior
	Euphoria	Agitation
	Sociability	Combative behavior
	Productivity	Dysphoria
	Mental clarity	Hallucinations
	Sexual arousal	Insomnia
	Sharpened awareness	Paranoia
		Psychosis
		Suicidal thoughts

Adapted from Miotto K, Striebel J, Cho AK, Wang C. Clinical and pharmacological aspects of bath salt use: A review of the literature and case reports. *Drug and Alcohol Dependence.* 2013; 132(1–2): 1–12.[31]

of federal prisoners reported being intoxicated at the time of their offenses.[35] Being under the influence of drugs or alcohol has been considered a substantial factor in crimes ranging from public intoxication and driving under the influence to theft crimes such as larceny, robbery, or burglary and violent crimes such as rape, assault, and murder.[36] Substance use itself is a significant predictive factor used in violence risk assessment.[37] Depending on the jurisdiction, possession of an intoxicating substance itself could be considered a crime.

Defenses Available for Crimes Committed During Intoxication

The Model Penal Code § 2.08 defines intoxication as "a disturbance of mental and or physical capabilities resulting from the introduction of substances into the body."[38] Our recently retired diagnostic system (*DSM-IV TR*) defined intoxication generically as "the development of a reversible substance-specific syndrome due to recent ingestion of (or exposure to) a substance . . . resulting in clinically significant maladaptive behavioral or psychological changes that are due to the effect of the substance on the central nervous system (e.g., belligerence, mood lability, cognitive impairment, impaired judgment, impaired social or occupational functioning) and develop during or shortly after use of the substance" (p. 199).[39] *DSM-5*, however, eschews a generic definition of intoxication in favor of descriptions of substance-specific intoxication syndromes.[40] Another authority defines intoxication as "a erversible syndrome caused by a specific substance (e.g., alcohol) that affects one or more of the following mental functions: memory, orientation, mood, judgment, and behavioral, social, or occupational functioning" (p. 384).[41]

Depending on jurisdiction, a defendant may be able to claim that voluntary (self-induced) intoxication negated the capacity to form specific criminal intent. A defendant may also claim involuntary or pathologic intoxication. Voluntary intoxication occurs when a person consumes a substance that is known to be intoxicating, usually for effect, without any coercion or duress. It should be noted that the person need not intend to become intoxicated. Involuntary intoxication, on the other hand, can include the consumption of an intoxicant as a result of coercion, deceit, or duress or even as a consequence of medical advice. In this case, the defendant would be claiming that the resulting behavior could not have been predicted—because someone poisoned the defendant, the effect was grossly in excess of what would reasonably have been expected, or the effect was not known to the defendant or to the community generally.

Across the United States, evidence of voluntary intoxication cannot be used either as an excuse for a crime or in the service of an insanity defense. There is also no constitutional right to use evidence of intoxication in one's defense. It may be used in specific-intent crimes in some jurisdictions, however, if the defendant can show inability to form the requisite intent under the influence of a substance. Such a tactic has the effect of creating reasonable doubt about the government's charge, while not precluding conviction on a lesser charge (e.g., failure to prove murder but conviction for manslaughter).

There are variants among jurisdictions of which expert witnesses must be aware. For example, in Pennsylvania, evidence of intoxication, when it negates specific intent, can reduce first-degree murder to a third-degree charge. Otherwise, such evidence is not admissible. Voluntary intoxication would not tend to be a defense in general-intent crimes—for example, those in which the element of culpability is recklessness. Temporary insanity or short-lived mental changes secondary to voluntary intoxication are not considered a mental disease or defect for the insanity defense but may result in a reduced verdict or sentence or in a finding of "guilty but mentally ill." However, persistent or "settled" insanity may be permitted if the mental state persists beyond the substance use (see below). Pathologic intoxication, a variant of involuntary intoxication, in which a person suffers intoxication grossly out of proportion to the amount of substance consumed, is a rarely used defense that may successfully be used for exculpation in first-time users.[36,42] Blackouts as a result of substance intoxication generally cannot be used successfully in a criminal defense. In those cases, while the presence of amnesia may imply intoxication, memory gaps per se do not indicate whether the defendant formed the requisite intent. Defendants claiming that their crimes were committed during a blackout must be suspected of malingering (faking amnesia).

INTOXICATION VIEWED UNDER THE LAW

Some commentators have observed that even though clinical understanding of addiction and intoxication has grown more sophisticated, the way the law deals with addiction, intoxication, and criminal responsibility has changed little over the centuries.[42,43] Criminal law uses the theory of tracing to justify punishment of crimes committed under intoxication: While the defendant may have lost impulse control while intoxicated, responsibility can be traced to the onset of voluntarily consuming the substance. This was the logic used in the landmark case *Powell v. Texas*[44] to uphold the defendant's conviction. Powell was arrested for public drunkenness and found guilty. He subsequently appealed, stating that punishing him for being a chronic alcoholic would be a cruel and unusual punishment. During cross-examination, his expert witness agreed that when the defendant was sober he knew the difference between right and wrong and also admitted that the defendant's act of taking the first drink in any given instance "is a voluntary exercise of his will." During a telling part of the cross-examination, the defendant himself acknowledged that he was able to prohibit himself from having no more than one drink the morning of the trial because he "was supposed to be here on trial."

Reviewing the law and literature on voluntary intoxication and criminal responsibility for the state of Hawaii, Carter-Yamauchi cited several moral/ legal theories of why self-induced states should not be given dispensation under the law.[45] First, she points out that the concept of insanity presumes that one acquires the condition involuntarily. The insanity defense rests on the presence of a "disease of the mind"; intoxication generally does not meet this standard. Thus, an artificial, voluntarily induced insanity—no matter how severe—would not be an excuse for criminal conduct. Second, the ingestion of substances is a manifestation of free will, notwithstanding the mounting evidence of addiction as a disease, or at least as a condition with serious biologic substrates.[46,47] Therefore, the substance user willingly accepts all the risks that flow from intoxication. Other arguments for strict liability include that the user is demonstrating immoral intent by getting intoxicated, that intoxication is a voluntary disavowal of reason and conscience, that intoxication is easily feigned, and that to permit intoxication as an excuse would deter prosecutions.

VOLUNTARY INTOXICATION

Persons who commit crimes while intoxicated characteristically say they did not mean to do it. Beyond this cliché, there are obviously individuals who are so intoxicated that they could not have formed the requisite criminal intent for the crime. Yet, they may have no recourse under the law of their jurisdiction. In cases of voluntary intoxication, statutes vary as to the applicability of *mens rea* (culpable mind) defenses. A 1999 review by Marlowe and colleagues lists 4 types of approaches to negation of *mens rea*.[48] About one fourth of jurisdictions bar such evidence outright. Twenty jurisdictions permit evidence of intoxication to negate an element of intent, although this would generally not apply to recklessness (e.g., drunk driving). About the same number of jurisdictions restrict the evidence to specific-intent crimes. In these states, the defendant would still be liable under a general-intent scenario. The fourth type, noted in 3 states, is the restriction of evidence of intoxication to first-degree murder, whereby negation of the higher elements of the offense (e.g., knowledge, purpose, premeditation, or deliberateness) would reduce the conviction to second or third degree. Marlowe and colleagues point out that, irrespective of the unpopularity of intoxication defenses, a defendant retains the right to raise the issue as mitigation in sentencing.[48] In our experience, such evidence can backfire, and one commentator has called it "counterintuitive."[49] As Justice Scalia pointed out in *Montana v. Egelhoff*,[50] evidence of intoxication has been used historically as an *aggravating* factor. Nevertheless, at a capital sentencing hearing, evidence of intoxication (or any mental health issue that would not rise to the level of a defense) can be employed in mitigation.[51,52]

INVOLUNTARY (PATHOLOGIC) INTOXICATION

In certain situations, a defendant demonstrates nonculpable behavior while intoxicated. These would include persons who were dosed surreptitiously or against their will, persons experiencing side effects of prescription drugs, and persons experiencing unexpected effects of substances taken in small amounts (pathologic intoxication). The defendant, having demonstrated the cause and extent of the intoxication, must then show that the intoxication caused a condition analogous to legal insanity. This makes the involuntary intoxication defense an affirmative (not simply a failure of proof of culpability) and complete (acquittal) defense when the facts support the test for insanity.[49] Operationally, an instance of involuntary intoxication is characterized by the individual's not exercising any volitional behavior or intent toward developing the intoxicated state. It is important to note that it is insufficient for a defendant to assert the mere presence of addiction in support of such a claim.[45]

INTOXICATION AND DUE PROCESS

States have taken action to reject voluntary-intoxication defenses. The intoxication defense was outlawed by the Montana legislature in 1987. Under the Montana statute, evidence of intoxication could not be used, even to negate an element of intent. Defendant Egelhoff sought to use evidence of intoxication at his murder trial, but it was barred. The Montana Supreme Court, however, reversed, citing the defendant's due process right to present a defense. Montana appealed to the U.S. Supreme Court, which ruled in 1996 that there is no fundamental right to use evidence of intoxication as a defense.[50] For example, Justice Scalia noted that common-law tradition did not permit a voluntary intoxication defense. At least 14 states followed Montana's approach, with several cases and statutes signaling a growing distaste for such defenses.[49] This is not to say that there is a constitutional ban on evidence of intoxication, only that states are not required to have them. On the contrary, about 80% of jurisdictions admit such evidence under certain circumstances.[48]

A defendant has a right at a capital sentencing proceeding to adduce any evidence of character that might be relevant.[51,52] Yet obstacles remain. Recently, the Supreme Court declined to review a ruling of the Fifth Circuit that rejected a capital defendant's argument that a Texas jury was not properly instructed on his alcohol abuse.[53] Specifically, the defendant said that the state's law was unconstitutional because it did not specifically identify alcohol abuse as a potential mitigating factor.

The Fifth Circuit noted that the Supreme Court in *Penry v. Lynaugh* established that a sentencing jury must be informed of severe mental retardation and abuse.[54] But in *Penry* this type of evidence was limited to that which demonstrates a "uniquely severe permanent handicap with which the defendant was burdened through no fault of his own," excluding alcoholism and intoxication at the time of the offense. Instead, the jury could have chosen to consider alcoholism under instructions to consider the deliberateness of the defendant's conduct and future dangerousness.

The Supreme Court also declined to review a similar ruling of the Fifth Circuit that dismissed a defendant's assertion that the Texas capital sentencing scheme was unconstitutional. The defendant argued that it did not specifically direct the jury to consider the mitigating evidence of his drug and alcohol use at the time of the offense, his history of drug and alcohol abuse, a long history of severe abuse as a child, a pattern of suicide attempts and substance abuse within his immediate family, and impairment of his mental, academic, social, and behavioral functioning.[55] Thus, it appears as if the usually wide-open approach to evidence of mental disorders at sentencing has its limitations, at least to the extent that there is no constitutional protection. Marlowe and colleagues' review found that 5 states admitted evidence of intoxication in sentencing, but the majority of jurisdictions either dealt with it on a case-by-case basis or have not addressed it.[48]

SETTLED INSANITY

While it is clear that voluntary intoxication and involuntary intoxication occupy their own domains and carry widely divergent implications, there is an acknowledgment within the law that the voluntary use of substances can lead to long-lasting or permanent mental effects.[45,48,56] Although it is difficult to define exactly where substance use ends and substance-induced persistent mental illness begins, some jurisdictions permit evidence of a "fixed" or "settled" insanity under the statutes for the insanity defense. A 1986 California case listed 4 criteria for the use of a settled insanity defense: (1) the insanity is fixed and stable; (2) the condition lasts for a reasonable period of time; (3) the condition is not solely dependent on the ingestion and duration of the drug; and (4) the defendant's state of mind meets the jurisdiction's legal test for insanity.[45,57] Under the federal Insanity Defense Reform Act, however, any taint of voluntary substance use negates the defense. Other jurisdictions have rejected settled insanity on moral or public policy grounds.[45]

Virginia permits a standard insanity defense (for psychotic disorders and mental retardation), an involuntary intoxication defense, as well as settled insanity and intoxication defenses in specific-intent offenses. In its criteria for settled insanity, the code calls for "organic impairment, with psychotic symptoms, resulting from long-term substance use." Citing a constitutional right to a psychiatric/psychological evaluation in preparation of an insanity defense, the Virginia code specifically endorses this right for indigent defendants who show "probable cause" to believe that sanity issues will be raised.[58] This is intriguing in light of the later Supreme Court ruling that there is no constitutional right for defendants to assert intoxication defenses.[50] It would appear that if there were a reasonable chance of reaching the criteria for insanity, the defendant would be at least able to be evaluated in this jurisdiction. Colorado, by contrast, rejected settled insanity defenses in 1993.[59] In *Bieber*, the defendant attempted to use medical evidence of amphetamine-induced delusional disorder to proffer an insanity defense. The defense was not permitted because the syndrome in question was derivative of the use of intoxicating substances. Moreover, since there is no temporary insanity provision in Colorado, the court could not make an exception for a drug-induced version of it, whether or not the condition persisted beyond the known limits of ordinary amphetamine intoxication. The U.S. Supreme Court declined to rule on *Bieber* and the question of the right to be tried by way of a settled insanity defense.

WHERE DO DESIGNER DRUGS FALL IN THIS PARADIGM?

It appears that several new designer drugs have quickly established significant use in the United States within a few years of their introduction. Given the dearth of epidemiologic data regarding their prevalence, we can only speculate on the use prevalence in the community. Whether many of these emerging designer drugs are just the latest fad in drug use or here for the long term remains to be seen. However, even with the assumption that the use of designer drugs, especially SCs and synthetic cathinones, will remain circumscribed, the rate of reported adverse neuropsychiatric effects remains quite high. Unlike other more established drugs, the collective user experience with respect to serious risks is only developing, and these synthetic substances are still attractive as "legal" alternatives that do not get detected as easily. And unlike their natural counterparts, SCs and synthetic cathinones are associated with a higher rate of behavioral effects such as anxiety, agitation, paranoia, auditory and visual hallucinations, combativeness, and aggression. A review of the literature suggests that many of these adverse effects seem to be completely unanticipated by users.[37] But does this render their effect involuntary, thereby relieving the user of responsibility? This will be the focal point of forensic testimony and should be anticipated by expert witnesses.

EXPERT WITNESS APPROACHES

Since there is no universal right to present defense testimony on intoxication, each expert must know the prevailing statutes and case law. There is also a strategic decision the defense attorney must make regarding framing the substance-related mental state as a specific substance-induced psychotic disorder, voluntary intoxication, or involuntary (pathologic) intoxication. This will determine the trajectory of the expert's report, whether on the defense or prosecution side. Defenses relying on negation of *mens rea* (voluntary intoxication) often have the advantage of creating reasonable doubt as to whether the criminal act was specifically intended; involuntary intoxication may have the additional burden of proving that the intoxicated state produced a version of insanity that must be proved by a preponderance or even clear and convincing evidence. The witness' report and testimony must show awareness of these subtleties and adjust the language accordingly.

For experts assisting the prosecution, the thrust of the government's argument would tend to be along the lines of construing the effects of the substance as voluntary. In that way, the defendant will more likely be viewed as accountable for the downstream effects of the intoxication, whether or not the result was anticipated. Of course, even experienced drug users do not set out to become psychotic and violent. A credible prosecution expert, therefore, will speak to the observed or inferred clinical effects of the substance and let the prosecutor argue, where applicable, that the condition does not conform to statutory defenses.

Psychiatric experts on either side have an obligation to explore aspects of the claim of intoxication. These include the following: substantiation that the defendant used a substance in a relevant time frame to the underlying offense; evidence of the nature of the substance; when possible, laboratory evidence of the substance; evidence of other substances or ongoing mental disorders affecting the defendant during the time in question; corroboration of the defendant's behavior; collateral evidence that the defendant's behavior represented a departure from usual; any evidence that the defendant was dosed or would not have been able to anticipate the effects of the substance; and an assessment of the defendant's knowledge and anticipated effects of the substance.

REFERENCES

1. Substance Abuse and Mental Health Services Administration. *Results from the 2011 National Survey on Drug Use and Health: Summary of National Findings.* Rockville, MD; 2012: 174.
2. Substance Abuse and Mental Health Services Administration. *Drug Abuse Warning Network, 2011: National Estimates of Drug-Related Emergency Department Visits.* August 5, 2013. Available online at http://www.samhsa.gov/data/2k13/DAWN2k11ED/DAWN2k11ED.htm.
3. Johnston LD, O'Malley PM, Bachman JG, Schulenberg JE. *Monitoring the Future National Results on Drug Use: 2012 Overview, Key Findings on Adolescent Drug Use.* Ann Arbor: Institute for Social Research, The University of Michigan; 2013.

4. American Association of Poison Control Centers. *Bath Salts Data*. August 5, 2013. Available online at https://aapcc.s3.amazonaws.com/files/library/Bath_Salts_Data_for_Website_7.31.2013.pdf.

5. Department of Justice NDIC. *Synthetic Cathinones (Bath Salts): An Emerging Domestic Threat*. 2011. Available online at http://www.justice.gov/archive/ndic/pubs44/44571/44571p.pdf.

6. Green N. The unraveling of Rudy Eugene, aka the Causeway face attacker. MiamiHerald.com, July 16, 2012. Available online at http://www.miamiherald.com/2012/07/14/2895973/the-unraveling-of-rudy-eugene.html.

7. Bryan S. Causeway Cannibal: Even experts question claim that Rudy Eugene was not on bath salts. *Sun Sentinel*, July 6, 2012; Available online at http://articles.sun-sentinel.com/2012-07-06/news/fl-bath-salts-tests-20120706_1_bath-salts-synthetic-marijuana-clandestine-labs.

8. Goodnough A. An alarming new stimulant, sold legally in many states. *New York Times*, July 17, 2011, p A1.

9. O'Malley DJ. Police: Man who stabbed priest was high on bath salts. March 10, 2011; Available online at http://thetimes-tribune.com/news/police-man-who-stabbed-priest-was-high-on-bath-salts-1.1116514.

10. Warren B. Snorting bath salts pushed St. Tammany man to suicide. January 16, 2011. Available online at http://www.nola.com/crime/index.ssf/2011/01/snorting_bath_salts_pushed_st.html.

11. Marder J. The drug that never lets go. *PBS NewsHour*, Sept. 20, 2012. Available online at http://www.pbs.org/newshour/multimedia/bath-salts/.

12. Clarridge C. Fort Lewis soldier who killed wife, self had taken synthetic "bath salts" drug. *Seattle Times*, June 13, 2011. Available onlinen at http://seattletimes.com/html/localnews/2015311562_bathsalts14m.html.

13. To The Maximus Foundation. 2themax.org.

14. Stackhouse TP. Regulators in Wackyland: capturing the last of the designer drugs. *Arizona Law Review*. 2012; 54: 1105–1157.

15. Kau G. Flashback to the Federal Analog Act of 1986: mixing rules and standards in the cauldron. *University of Pennsylvania Law Review*. 2008; 156(4): 1077–1115.

16. U.S.C. Title 21—FOOD AND DRUGS. 2013.

17. *U.S.* v. *Klecker*, 348 F.3d 69 (2003).

18. Federal Register/Vol. 76, No. 40/Tuesday, March 1, 2011.

19. Moran JH. Smart resource allocation needed to study "legal highs." *Nature Medicine*. 2011; 17(11): 1339. doi:10.1038/nm1111-1339.

20. Vardakou I, Pistos C, Spiliopoulou C. Spice drugs as a new trend: mode of action, identification and legislation. *Toxicol Lett*. 2010; 197(3): 157–162.

21. Fattore L, Fratta W. Beyond THC: the new generation of cannabinoid designer drugs. *Front Behav Neurosci*. 2011; 5: 60. Available online at http://www.ncbi.nlm.nih.gov/pmc/articles/PMC3187647/#__ffn_sectitle.

22. Auwarter V, Dresen S, Weinmann W, Muller M, Putz M, Ferreiros N. "Spice" and other herbal blends: harmless incense or cannabinoid designer drugs? *J Mass Spectrometry*. 2009; 44(5): 832–837.

23. Wiley JL, Marusich JA, Huffman JW, Balster RL, Thomas BF. Hijacking of basic research: the case of synthetic cannabinoids. *Methods Rep RTI Press*, November 2011. Available online at http://www.ncbi.nlm.nih.gov/pmc/articles/PMC3567606/

24. Atwood BK, Lee D, Straiker A, Widlanski TS, Mackie K. CP47,497-C8 and JWH073, commonly found in "Spice" herbal blends, are potent and efficacious CB(1) cannabinoid receptor agonists. *Eur J Pharmacol.* 2011; 659(2–3): 139–145.

25. Uchiyama N, Kikura-Hanajiri R, Ogata J, Goda Y. Chemical analysis of synthetic cannabinoids as designer drugs in herbal products. *Forensic Sci Intl.* 2010; 198(1–3): 31–38.

26. Zuardi AW, Shirakawa I, Finkelfarb E, Karniol IG. Action of cannabidiol on the anxiety and other effects produced by delta 9-THC in normal subjects. *Psychopharmacology.* 1982; 76(3): 245–250.

27. Caulkins JP. *Marijuana Legalization: What Everyone Needs to Know.* New York: Oxford University Press; 2012.

28. Seely KA, Lapoint J, Moran JH, Fattore L. Spice drugs are more than harmless herbal blends: a review of the pharmacology and toxicology of synthetic cannabinoids. *Progr Neuropsychopharmacol Biol Psychiatry.* 2012; 39(2): 234–243.

29. Zawilska JB, Wojcieszak J. Designer cathinones: an emerging class of novel recreational drugs. *Forensic Sci Intl.* 2013; 231(1–3): 42–53.

30. Carroll FI, Lewin AH, Mascarella SW, Seltzman HH, Reddy PA. Designer drugs: a medicinal chemistry perspective. *Ann NY Acad Sci.* 2012; 1248: 18–38.

31. Miotto K, Striebel J, Cho AK, Wang C. Clinical and pharmacological aspects of bath salt use: a review of the literature and case reports. *Drug Alcohol Depen.* 2013; 132(1–2): 1–12.

32. Shanks KG, Dahn T, Behonick G, Terrell A. Analysis of first- and second-generation legal highs for synthetic cannabinoids and synthetic stimulants by ultra-performance liquid chromatography and time of flight mass spectrometry. *J Anal Toxicol.* 2012; 36(6): 360–371.

33. Aarde SM, Huang PK, Creehan KM, Dickerson TJ, Taffe MA. The novel recreational drug 3,4-methylenedioxypyrovalerone (MDPV) is a potent psychomotor stimulant: self-administration and locomotor activity in rats. *Neuropharmacology.* 2013; 71: 130–140.

34. Warrick BJ, Hill M, Hekman K, et al. A 9-state analysis of designer stimulant, "bath salt," hospital visits reported to poison control centers. *Ann Emerg Med.* 2013; 62(3): 244–251.

35. Karberg JC, James DJ. *Substance Dependence, Abuse, and Treatment of Jail Inmates, 2002.* Washington, DC: U.S. Department of Justice, Office of Justice Programs, Bureau of Justice Statistics; 2005.

36. Miller NS. *Principles of Addictions and the Law: Applications in Forensic, Mental Health, and Medical Practice.* Waltham, MA: Academic Press; 2010.

37. Fazel S, Langstrom N, Hjern A, Grann M, Lichtenstein P. Schizophrenia, substance abuse, and violent crime. *JAMA.* 2009; 301(19): 2016–2023.

38. American Bar Association. *Model Penal Code.* Philadelphia, American Law Institute, 1960: 349.

39. American Psychiatric Association. *Diagnostic and Statistical Manual of Mental Disorders: DSM-IV-TR (Text Revision),* 4th ed. Washington, DC: American Psychiatric Association; 2000.

40. American Psychiatric Association. *Diagnostic and Statistical Manual of Mental Disorders: DSM-5,* 5th ed. Washington, DC: American Psychiatric Publishing; 2013.

41. Sadock BJ, Kaplan HI, Sadock VA. *Kaplan & Sadock's Synopsis of Psychiatry,* 10th ed. Philadelphia: Lippincott Williams & Wilkins; 2007.

42. Weiss KJ. Wet and wild: PCP and criminal responsibility. *J Psychiatry Law.* 2004; 32: 361–384.
43. Murray PE. In need of a fix: reforming criminal law in light of a contemporary understanding of drug addiction. *UCLA Law Review.* 2013; 60: 1006–1046.
44. *Powell* v. *Texas*, 392 U.S. 514 (1968).
45. Carter-Yamauchi CA. *Drugs, Alcohol, and the Insanity Defense: The Debate Over "Settled" Insanity.* Honolulu, HI: Legislative Reference Bureau; 1998.
46. Frances M, Frosch WA, Galanter M, et al. Responsibility and choice in addiction. *Psychiatric Serv.* 2002; 53: 707–713,
47. Ballantyne JC, Mao J. Opioid therapy for chronic pain. *N Engl J Med.* 2003; 349(20): 1943–1953.
48. Marlowe DB, Lambert JB, Thompson RG. Voluntary intoxication and criminal responsibility. *Behav Sci Law.* 1999; 17(2): 195–217.
49. Ingle MP. Law on the rocks: the intoxication defenses are being eighty-sixed. *Vanderbilt Law Review.* 2002; 55: 607–646.
50. *Montana* v. *Egelhoff*, 518 U.S. 37 (1996).
51. *Lockett* v. *Ohio*, 438 U.S. 586 (1978).
52. *Eddings* v. *Oklahoma*, 455 U.S. 104 (1982).
53. *Harris* v. *Cockrell*, 535 U.S. 958 (2002).
54. *Penry* v. *Lynaugh*, 492 U.S. 302 (1989).
55. *Miniel* v. *Cockrell*, 339 F. 3d 331 (2003).
56. Meloy JR. Voluntary intoxication and the insanity defense. *J Psychiatry Law.* 1992; 20: 439–457.
57. *People* v. *Skinner*, 241 Cal. App. 2d 752 (1986).
58. *Ake* v. *Oklahoma*, 470 U.S. 68 (1985).
59. *Bieber* v. *People*, 835 P.2d 542 (Colo. App. 1992).

INDEX

from gunshot wound, PET admissibility, 127
TBI (traumatic brain injury), 137–138, 145–146
See also CTE (chronic traumatic encephalopathy)
brain development, effects of stress
childhood maltreatment, 47–54
considerations in sentencing and mitigation, 59–60
implications for juvenile offenders, 60–61
neuroscience of, 54–59
See also PTSD (posttraumatic stress disorder)
brain imaging. *See* neuroimaging; nuclear medicine imaging.
brain scans. *See* neuroimaging; nuclear medicine imaging.
Brody, Anita, 142
burden of proof, 1
Burgess, R. v., 111
Burr, State of New Jersey v., 75–76, 77

Caddell, State v., 113
California v. Larsen, 76
Canada, parasomnia cases, 111
Caro, Fernando, 131
Carrizalez, Miguel, 127
Carter-Yamauchi, C. A., 163
Causeway face attacker, 156–157
childhood disintegrative disorder. *See* ASD (autism spectrum disorder).
childhood maltreatment
and criminal offending, 50–51
misconceptions of, 47
rates of, 50
risk for adult criminal behavior, 51
risk for juvenile delinquency, 51
See also ACE (Adverse Childhood Experience) Study; adverse childhood experiences
childhood maltreatment, trauma
vs. adverse experience, 48
definition, 47
vs. PTSD, 49–50
childhood memory, 36–38
children. *See* adolescent; childhood.
child sexual abuse accommodation syndrome (CSAAS). *See* CSAAS

(child sexual abuse accommodation syndrome).
child sexual abuse investigation
characteristics of abuse, 31
childhood memory, 36–38
coaching for false allegations, 38
credibility of child witnesses, 31
delayed disclosure, 32
ecological validity, 41
entrapment, 32
episodic memory, 36–37
evidence base for testimony, 38–41
external validity, 41
false report rate, 34–35
forensic interviewing protocols, 38–41
helplessness, 31–32
limits on testimony, 41
loss of family support, 32
memory retrieval, 37
power assertion, 32
recanting, 35
research on children's disclosure, 34–35
retracting allegations, 32–33
secrecy, 31–32
semantic memory, 36–37
suggestibility, 36–38
See also CSAAS (child sexual abuse accommodation syndrome)
China, lie detection, 84
chronic traumatic encephalopathy (CTE). *See* CTE (chronic traumatic encephalopathy).
Clearwater, A. T., 4
Cloud Nine. *See* synthetic cathinones (bath salts).
coaching children for false allegations, 38
cognitive control brain system, 16
confidentiality, ethics of forensic psychiatry, xviii
confusional arousals, 106
Controlled Substance Analogue Act of 1986 (Federal Analog Act), 157–158
Controlled Substances Act of 1970 (CSA), 157–158
cool cognition, 17

intoxication
   defenses for crimes committed during, 161–162
   definition, 161–162
   from designer drugs, 167
   and due process, 165–166
   expert witness approaches, 167
   involuntary (pathologic), 164–165
   as a legal defense, 165–166
   legal view of, 163–164
   mens rea (guilty intent) defenses, 168
   settled insanity defense, 166–167
   voluntary, 162–163, 164
involuntary (pathologic) intoxication, 164–165
Ivory Coast. *See* synthetic cathinones (bath salts).
Ivory Snow. *See* synthetic cathinones (bath salts).
Ivory Wave. *See* synthetic cathinones (bath salts).

Jackson v. Hobbs, 19
Jiang, W., 95
Jones, P., 146
Jung, C. G., xv
juvenile court applications, adverse childhood experiences, 60–61
juvenile delinquency, role of childhood maltreatment, 51
juvenile offenders. *See* adolescent offenders.

K2. *See* SCs (synthetic cannabinoids).
Kalbe, E., 78
Kandel. E. R., 47–48
Kanner, Leo, 67
kidnapping by cesarean section, PET admissibility, 126–127
Kieczykowski, Adam, 114
Kiehl, Kent, 91–92
Korngold, C., 142
Kozel, Andrew, 86, 90
Kumho Tire Co., Ltd v. Carmichael, 8

Laken, Steven, 92
Langleben, Daniel, 86
Larsen, California v., 76
law of evidence, 1–2
learning, role of the mind, 47–48

legal citations. *See specific cases.*
legislation, Insanity Defense Reform Act of 1984, xiv
lie detection
   among Bedouins in Arabia, 84
   among psychopaths, xv
   in ancient China, 84
   hypnosis, xv
   a legal perspective, 96–97
   narcosis (truth serum), xv
   polygraphs, xv, 85
   during the Spanish Inquisition, 84
   through neuroimaging. *See* fMRI (functional magnetic resonance imaging).
life-course-persistent offenders, 21, 23
Lockett v. Ohio, 130
loss of family support, child sex abuse investigation, 32
Luedecke, Jan, 112–113
Lynn, William, 33

Mahoney, Mark, 68
maltreatment of children. *See* childhood maltreatment.
Mansfield, Lord, 3–4
Marcus, D. K., 128–129
Marston, William, 5
Martin, L., 114–115
Martland, Harrison S., 136
maternal behavior
   in animals, 56–57
   in humans, 57–59
McClain v. Indiana, 112–113
McCollum, Darius, 69
McGowan, P. O., 57
McKinnon, Gary, 72, 77
memory
   childhood, 36–38
   episodic, 36–37
   retrieval, 37
   semantic, 36–37
mens rea (guilty intent)
   ASD defense in court, 73–74
   defense in nuclear medicine imaging case, 128–130
   definition, 110
   intoxication defense, 168
   parasomnias and criminal actions, 110–111

slow-wave sleep, 105
Smith v. Grant, xiv
Smith v. Mullin, 132
socioemotional brain system, 16
soldiers and veterans, CTE, 145– 146
somnambulism (sleepwalking)
    alcohol-induced, 113– 114
    description, 107
    history of, 102– 103, 112
    and insanity, 112– 113
    legal defense for, 111– 113
Spanish Inquisition, lie detection, 84
SPECT (single photon emission com-
        puted tomography)
    in capital murder trials, 132
    in nuclear medicine imaging,
        123– 124
    in support of diminished actuality, 130
Spence, Sean, 86
Spice. *See* SCs (synthetic cannabinoids).
State of New Jersey v. Burr, 75– 76, 77
State v. Caddell, 113
Steinberg, Steven, 114– 115
Step Wise Interview, 38
Stinnett, Bobbie Jo, 126– 127
stress, and brain development
    childhood maltreatment, 47– 54
    considerations in sentencing and
        mitigation, 59– 60
    implications for juvenile offenders,
        60– 61
    neuroscience of, 54– 59
    See also PTSD (posttraumatic stress
        disorder)
Strickland v. Washington, 131
substance use
    annual surveys, 155– 156
    current trends, 155– 156
    See also intoxication; SCs (synthetic
        cannabinoids); synthetic cathi-
        nones (bath salts)
suggestibility, child sexual abuse, 36– 38
suggestiveness, minimizing during
        interviews, 40
Sullivan v. Florida, 19
Summit, R. C., 31, 33
synthetic cannabinoids (SCs). *See* SCs
        (synthetic cannabinoids).
synthetic cathinones (bath salts)
    adverse clinical effects, 160

description, 159– 160
main ingredients, 159
neuropsychiatric effects of, 161
physical effects of, 161
prevalence of, 156
See also SCs (synthetic cannabinoids)
Synthetic Drug Abuse Prevention Act of
    2012 (SDAPA), 158

TBI (traumatic brain injury), 137– 138,
    145– 146. *See also* CTE (chronic
    traumatic encephalopathy).
tDCS (transcranial direct current
    stimulation), 89
teens. *See* adolescent.
Tennard v. Dretke, 130
testimony of expert witnesses.
    See expert testimony; expert
    witnesses.
TF-CBT (trauma-focused cognitive
    behavior therapy), 60
the jury system, expert witnesses *vs.*, xiv
therapy
    for adverse childhood experiences, 60
    TF-CBT (trauma-focused cognitive
        behavior therapy), 60
Thomas, Clarence, on lie detection,
    96– 97
Tibbs v. Commonwealth, 113
timing of lie detection tests, 95– 96
Tirrell, Albert, 112
ToM (Theory of Mind), 70, 77– 78
transcranial direct current stimulation
    (tDCS), 89
trauma
    vs. adverse experience, 48
    definition, 47
    vs. PTSD, 49– 50
trauma-focused cognitive behavior
    therapy (TF-CBT), 60
traumatic brain injury (TBI), 137– 138,
    145– 146. *See also* CTE (chronic
    traumatic encephalopathy).
*A Treatise on the Medical Jurisprudence of
    Insanity*, xiii, 103
trials
    excluding evidence, 125
    motion in limine, 125
    phases of, 124, 133
    sentencing. *See* criminal sentencing.